MARINE CORPS Daily 16 Workouts

MARINE CORPS Daily 16 Workouts

Marine Fitness
for the Civilian Athlete

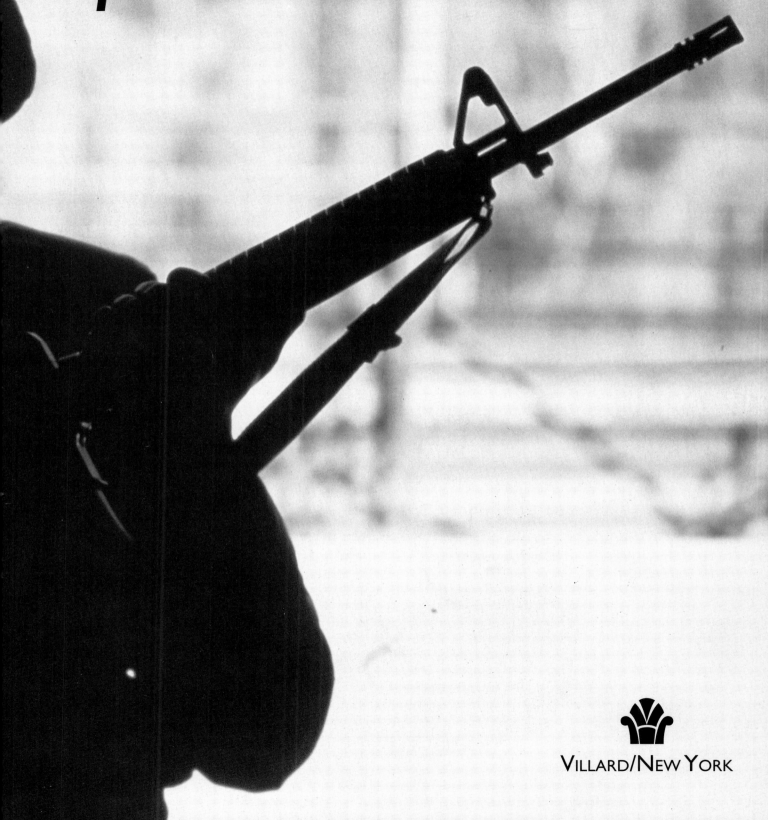

VILLARD/NEW YORK

ACKNOWLEDGMENTS

On behalf of Freundlich Communications, which compiled, edited, and packaged the *Marine Corps Daily 16 Workouts,* I would like to thank the following people.

John Korper's love of Marine Corps tradition and his dedication and loyalty to this project will always be dear to me. To Martina Nicholls, who at the start of this project cleared my path to Harlan Ullman, former Navy lieutenant commander and professor at the Naval War College. Mr. Ullman introduced me to his friends at the highest level of the Marine Corps cadre, and this project would not have gotten off the ground without him. Thanks to former Marine commandant, General Carl E. Mundy, Jr., for his early backing, and to General Thomas Morgan, Lieutenant General Anthony Lukeman, and Major General L. M. Palm, all retired, and allies of the Marine Corps Association in Quantico, Virginia, who spent long hours seeing that my access to the right sources and venues was facilitated. Thanks to Brigadier General K. T. Holcomb, director, Training and Education Division, USMC, for his support and for leading me to Lieutenant Colonel Leon Pappa, who cleared the way for my visit to Parris Island. And, finally, thanks to the drill instructors (especially Ken) at Parris Island, who patiently answered my questions, taught me the Daily 16, and let me watch their recruits in action.

–Lawrence S. Freundlich

Library of Congress Cataloging-in-Publication Data

Marine Corps Daily 16 Workouts: Marine fitness for the civilian athlete [Freundlich Communications].
    p. cm.
  ISBN 0-375-75132-7
  1. Exercise.   2. Physical fitness.   3. United States Marine Corps   I. Freundlich Communications
GV481.M373   1999
613.7'1—dc21 98-15283

Packaged by Freundlich Communications, Inc.
333 East 30th Street
New York, NY 10016

Designed by Tony Meisel

Random House website address: www.atrandom.com
Printed in the United States of America on acid-free paper
98765432
First Edition

Contents

Introduction

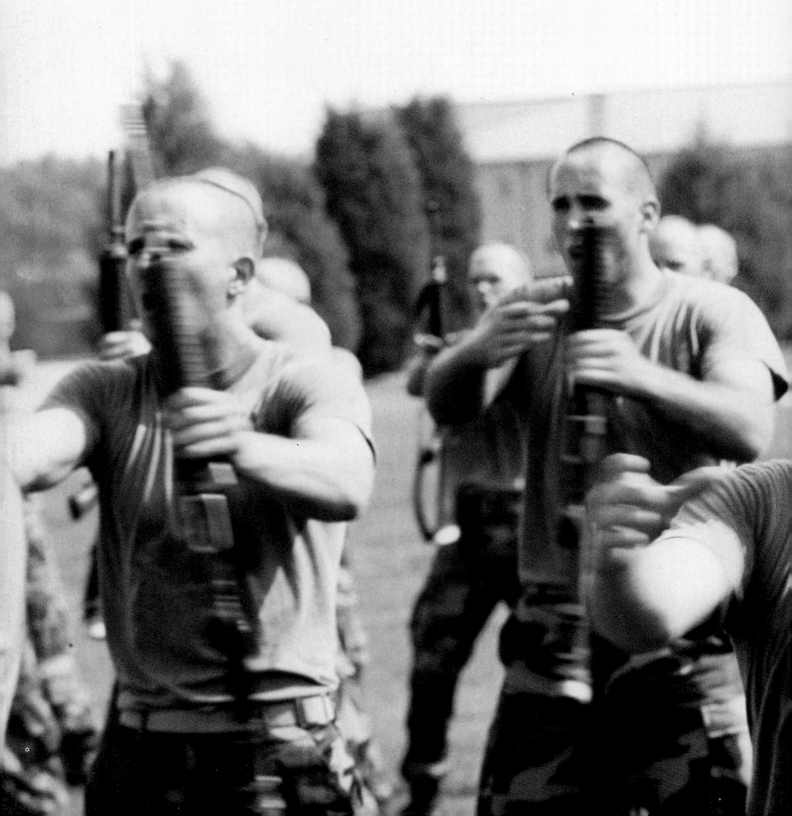

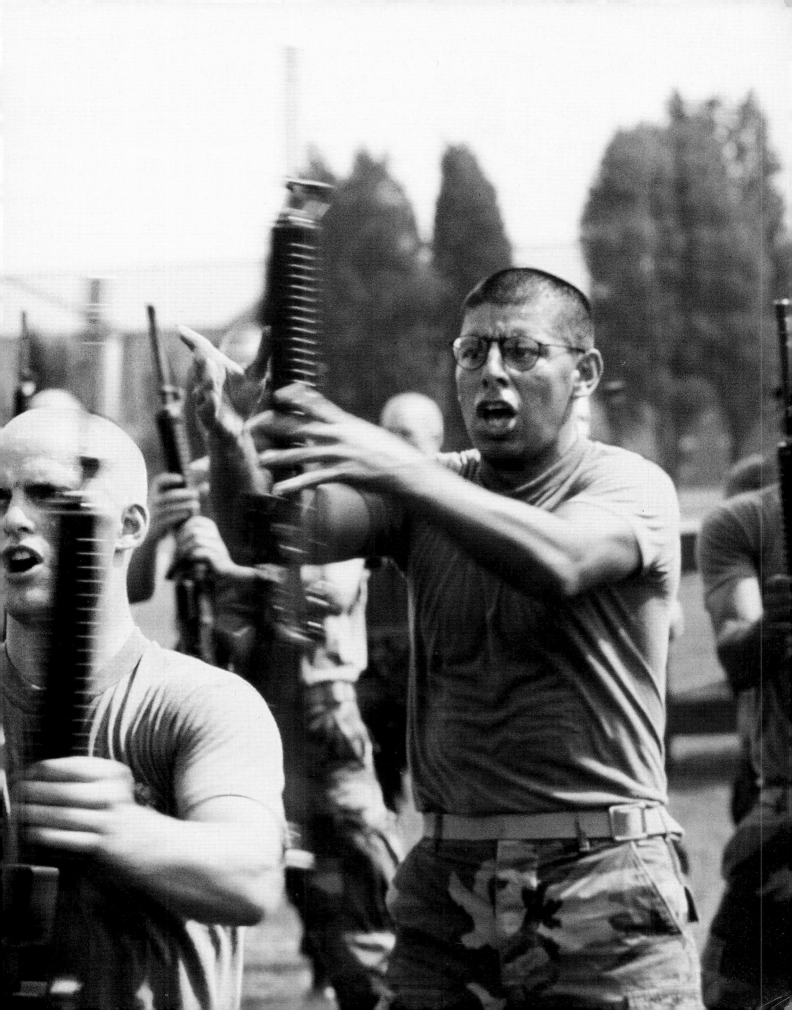

NOTE TO READERS

This is a rigorous exercise program. Neither the Author nor the Publisher can assume responsibility for risks associated with engaging in the activities described in this book. Each individual is responsible for determining if he or she is fit enough to undertake the rigors of the Daily 16 calisthenics program. As with any exercise program, before starting the Daily 16 and individual should consult his physician or health care practitioner and take into account any special medical conditions or limitations he may have. The goal of this program is to achieve peak physical conditioning without causing new injuries or exacerbating existing ones. Each individual is responsible for knowing her own limitations and taking appropriate steps to protect herself from exercise-related injuries.

Introduction

Most people associate the physical excellence of Marines with the dramatic capabilities they show in combat. They slither under barbed wire with live ammo firing overhead; they rappel down ropes from perilous heights; they are deadly in hand-to-hand combat; they leap from helicopters into jungle terrain; they storm beaches in heavy seas, laden with the weight of their weapons; they march many miles in tropical heat, carrying more than 50 pounds of equipment; they carry wounded comrades to safety.

Every Marine, male and female, who passes muster in recruit training must be able to perform these harsh and taxing maneuvers, and the reason he/she can rests on the foundation of the physical fitness training each has satisfactorily completed during basic training.

When Marine recruits arrive at either one of our two training depots in San Diego, California, or Parris Island, South Carolina, they face the prospect of having to live up to one of the strictest physical training regimens known to any military service. Under the aggressive and no-nonsense discipline of their Marine drill instructors, these 17- to 28-year-old recruits will, in the course of 11 weeks, be shaped into strong, agile, combat-ready Marines.

At the center of the physical training process lies the Daily 16, a regimen of stretching, warm-up, and calisthenics exercises, which when augmented by a program of aerobic running and conditioning, gives the Marine recruits strength, endurance, agility, and quickness.

The Daily 16 and the running program that complements it can be followed by all dedicated men and women from teenagers to senior citizens who seek to be in admirable shape.

The terrain in which recruits train has been specially designed to make them combat-ready Marines. Recruits have access to large fields, running tracks, circuit and obstacle courses, and all sorts of equipment specifically designed for their military preparation.

These conditions are unlikely to be readily available to the civilian athlete. Therefore, circuit and obstacle courses have been eliminated, as have exercises that require swimming. However, you will find here time-tested physical training substitutions for these activities, which, if you are not actually training to be a Marine, will get you in the same kind of excellent shape a recruit must achieve. Along with the Daily 16, the running and treadmill aerobics perfected by Kenneth H. Cooper at his famous Cooper Institute for Aerobics Research, considered Marine Corps baseline guides for aerobic fitness, are key to a Daily 16 conditioning program under the familiar restrictions of city living, full-time occupations, and even retirement.

Major General L. M. Palm, U.S. Marine Corps (Ret.)
Executive Director, Marine Corps Association, Quantico, Virginia

The Daily 16

The Daily 16 is the calisthenics program at the heart of Marine Recruit Training, and, as of July 15, 1998, replaced the Daily 7, which had been used by the Marine Corps for many years. The Naval Health Research Center (NHRC) found that the Daily 7 tended to overemphasize upper body muscles and failed to target most lower body muscles. The NHRC also considered that some of the Daily 7 exercises were likely to produce injury. As evidence pointed to the need for a change, the NHRC developed the Daily 16 program, which stresses the importance of a proper warm-up and cool-down—one that includes light activity, mobility exercises, and flexibility training.

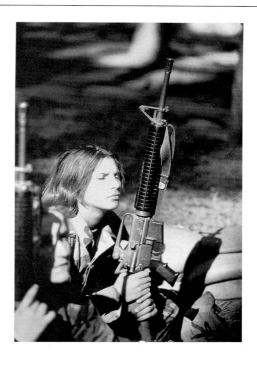

The Daily 16 always includes:
1. Dynamic Stretches, followed by
2. Static Stretches, followed by
3. Conditioning Exercises, followed by
4. Conditioning Runs, followed by
5. Cool-down, followed by
6. Conditioning Exercises, followed by
7. Static Stretches

Each Daily 16 routine takes about an hour, and there are a minimum of three Daily 16 workouts per week. Each of the routines in the Daily 16, e.g., "Dynamic Stretches," "Static Stretches," etc., is described on what the Marine Drill Instructors call their workout "Cards." To add variety to the Static Stretches and the Conditioning Exercises, there are 3 Static Stretches Cards (A, B, C) and 2 Conditioning Exercise Cards (1, 2). The Cards in each of these categories repeat some of the exercises of the previous card and also introduce some new routines. On exercise day #1, perform all the exercises on the first Card; on the next exercise day, do the exercises on the next Card in the exercise category.

HOW THE DAILY 16 IS PERFORMED
Always begin with a warmup consisting of 8 Dynamic Stretches which are held for 10 seconds. In performing all elements of the Daily 16, there is no break between each exercise, and no break between one Card and the next. This continuity is vital to achieving the aerobic and strengthening benefits of the program.

The Dynamic Stretches are followed immediately by 8 Static Stretches, each of which is held about 15 seconds.

Once the Static Stretches have been performed, a series of 8 Conditioning Calisthenics exercises is done beginning with 5 repetitions and increasing as training progresses. It would be reasonable to add one repetition for each 3 weeks of training until a comfortable maximum has been reached.

The next part of the workout involves running. In the first few weeks of training, the goal is to achieve a satisfactory aerobic base. By referring to the Aerobics Charts, the exerciser can measure his progress toward "good" condition and beyond. A satisfactory rating on these Cooper Charts should give you confidence that you are in satisfactory aerobic condition. While Marine recruits incorporate obstacle and circuit course training and swimming into their physical training sessions, these routines are, for reasons of practicality, not included here, and are not necessary in order to reach excellent levels of fitness within the Daily 16 program.

Once the run has been completed, the exerciser will enter the Cool-down period. First he/she will rehydrate by drinking at least one pint of water. After a slow walk he/she will do at least 5 more repetitions from the Conditioning Exercises followed by 8 more Static Stretches, which will be held for at least 30 seconds, or twice as long as in the Warm-up period.

Because recruits at the completion of their basic training will be required to pass a physical test including situps, chinups (and for females, flexed-armed hangs), a recruit at the end of each Daily 16 workout does the maximum number of these exercises he/she can. These exercises are described on pages 138-144.

FARTLEK

Once the civilian exerciser reaches satisfactory aerobic fitness as measured on the Cooper Charts, an additional day of exercise is added to the 3 days per week of the Daily 16. The Marines call their interval running and conditioning routine Fartlek training.

After reaching at least a satisfactory Cooper aerobic fitness level, another element is added. Once a week, the exerciser will run 220 yards (in the open or on a treadmill), then perform at least 5 repetitions of the Conditioning Calisthenics exercises, continuing until a full set of 8 exercises and running intervals is completed.

The advanced exerciser will progress to 3 miles or more of running, with the intervals between conditioning exercises stretched to 440 yards.

Remember, the running pace should conform to the fitness levels described on the Aerobic Charts. No exerciser should exceed the distance and the speed limits of his/her fitness category until he/she has performed for at least one week at the previous fitness level, and no Fartlek training should be performed until satisfactory aerobic fitness per age category has been attained.

SAMPLE MINIMUM FARTLEK WORKOUT FOR AEROBICALLY FIT AGE 40-49
Running distance: 2 miles
Running intervals: 220 yards or 1.25 miles
Running speed: 8 mph
Conditioning Exercises from Exercise Card 1: 5 repetitions

THE FARTLEK WORKOUT SEQUENCE
1. Warm-up and Dynamic Stretches
2. Static Stretches
3. Fartlek Intervals: Run › Wide pushups › Run › Donkey kicks › Run ›
   Dive bomber pushups › Run › Dirty dogs › Run › Side crunches › Run ›
   Lunges › Run › Side straddle hops
4. Cool-down
5. Dynamic stretches

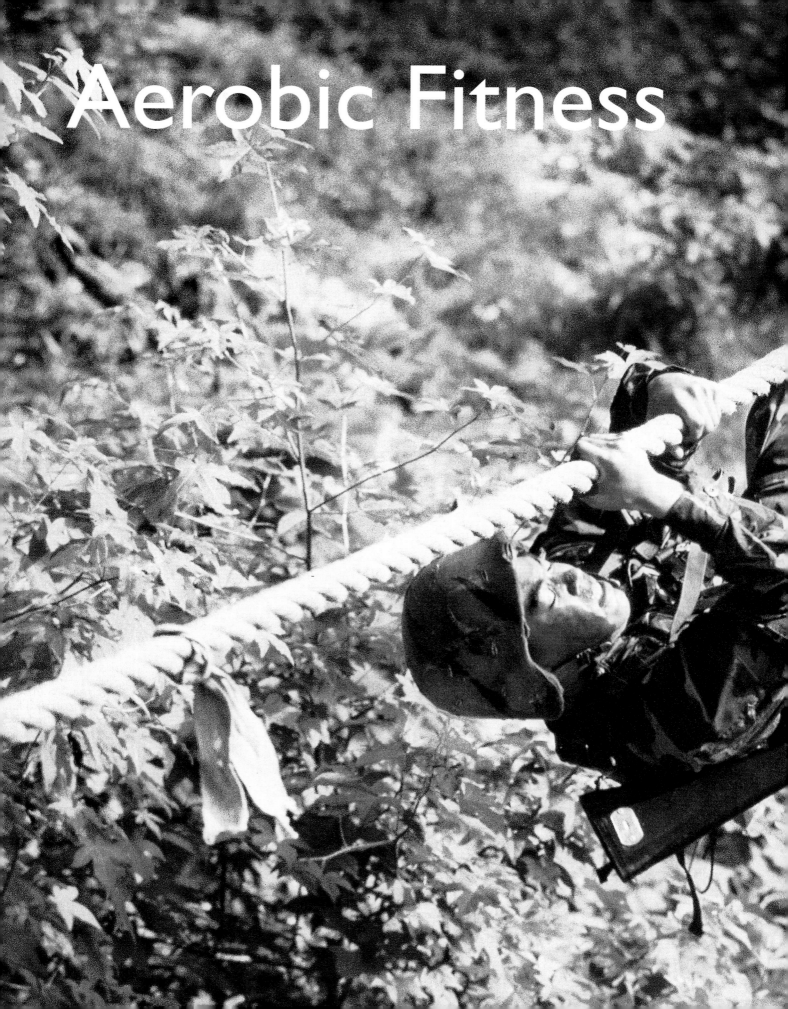

Aerobic Fitness

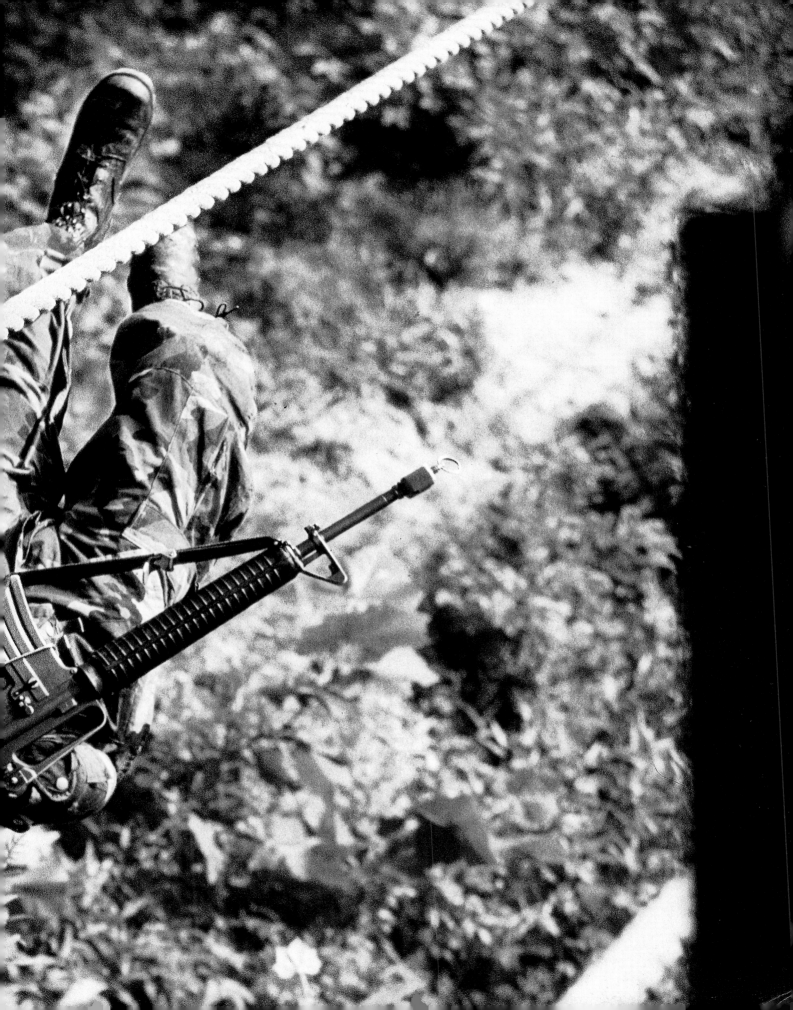

Aerobic Fitness

Dr. Kenneth H. Cooper is the pioneer of aerobic fitness conditioning and has been an invaluable consultant to the Marine Corps. The tests he has devised at his Cooper Institute for Aerobic Research are widely considered the standard measures of aerobic fitness. While Marine recruits run with their platoons outdoors on spacious fields, the civilian exerciser probably will be running in a gym or on a treadmill. Therefore, we have provided both outdoor aerobic fitness categories and their Cooper equivalents on progressive treadmill workouts.

Cooper assigns points according to the exerciser's ability to run at certain speeds and duration. He also provides age-related charts for both jogging and treadmill aerobic exercise programs that in a certain number of weeks bring the exerciser to at least satisfactory levels of aerobic conditioning.

	Average Points Per Week	
COOPER FITNESS CLASSIFICATIONS	Men	Women
Very Poor	less than 10	less than 8
Poor	10-20	8-15
Fair	21-31	16-26
Good	32-50	27-40
Excellent	51-74	41-64
Superior	75+	65+

COOPER DEFINITIONS FOR WALKING, JOGGING, RUNNING

Activity	Time/Mile
Walk	14:01 min. or longer
Walk-Jog	12:01-14:00 min.
Jog	9:00-12:00 min.
Run	under 9:00 min.

The Cooper Exercise Program by Age for Jogging and Progressive Treadmill

RUNNING/JOGGING EERCISE PROGRAM: UNDER 30 YEARS OF AGE

Week	Activity	Distance (miles)	Time Goal (min.)	Freq./Wk.	Points/Wk.
1	walk	2.0	32:00	3	13.5
2	walk	3.0	48:00	3	21.7
3	walk/jog	2.0	26:00	4	24.9
4	walk/jog	2.0	24:00	4	28.0
5	jog	2.0	22:00	4	31.6
6*	jog	2.0	20:00	4	36.0
7	jog	2.5	25:00	4	46.0
8	jog	2.5	23:00	4	49.5
9	jog	3.0	30:00	4	56.0
10	jog	3.0	27:00	4	61.3

*By the sixth week, a minimum aerobic fitness level has been reached (36 aerobic points per week), but it is suggested that a higher level of fitness be achieved. By the tenth week of the above program, a total of 61 points per week is being earned, consistent with the excellent category of aerobic fitness.

PROGRESSIVE TREADMILL EXERCISE PROGRAM: UNDER 30 YEARS OF AGE

Week	Activity	Treadmill Speed (mph)	Incline (%)	Time (min.)	Freq./Wk.	Points/Wk.
1	walk	4	flat	20:00	4	12.0
2	walk	4	flat	30:00	4	20.0
3	walk	4.5	flat	30:00	4	27.5
4	walk	4.5	5%	25:00	4	24.4
5*	walk/jog	5.0	flat	30:00	4	36.0
6	walk/jog	5.0	5%	25:00	4	32.2
7	jog	5.5	flat	30:00	4	45.5
8	jog	5.5	5%	25:00	4	41.0
9	jog	6.0	flat	30:00	4	56.0
10	jog	6.0	5%	30:00	4	61.6

*By the fifth week, adequate aerobic fitness has been reached (36 aerobic points per week) and it is permissible to continue at the exercise level.

By the tenth week, the excellent category has been achieved (61.6 aerobic points per week). Other combinations of speed, incline, duration, and frequency per week can be used to maintain the good or excellent fitness categories.

RUNNING/JOGGING EXERCISE PROGRAM: 30-49 YEARS OF AGE

Week	Activity	Distance (miles)	Time Goal (min.)	Freq./Wk.	Points/Wk.
1	walk	2.0	34:00	3	12.2
2	walk	2.5	42:00	3	16.3
3	walk	3.0	50:00	3	20.4
4	walk/jog	2.0	25:00	4	26.4
5	walk/jog	2.0	24:00	4	28.0
6	jog	2.0	22:00	4	31.6
7*	jog	2.0	20:00	4	36.0
8	jog	2.5	26:00	4	43.7
9	jog	2.5	25:00	4	46.0
10	jog	3.0	31:00	4	53.7
11	jog	3.0	29:00	4	57.6
12	jog	3.0	27:00	4	61.3

*By the seventh week, a minimum aerobic fitness level has been reached (36 aerobic points per week) but it is suggested that a higher level of fitness be achieved. By the twelfth week of the above program, a total of 61 points per week is being earned, consistent with the excellent category of aerobic fitness.

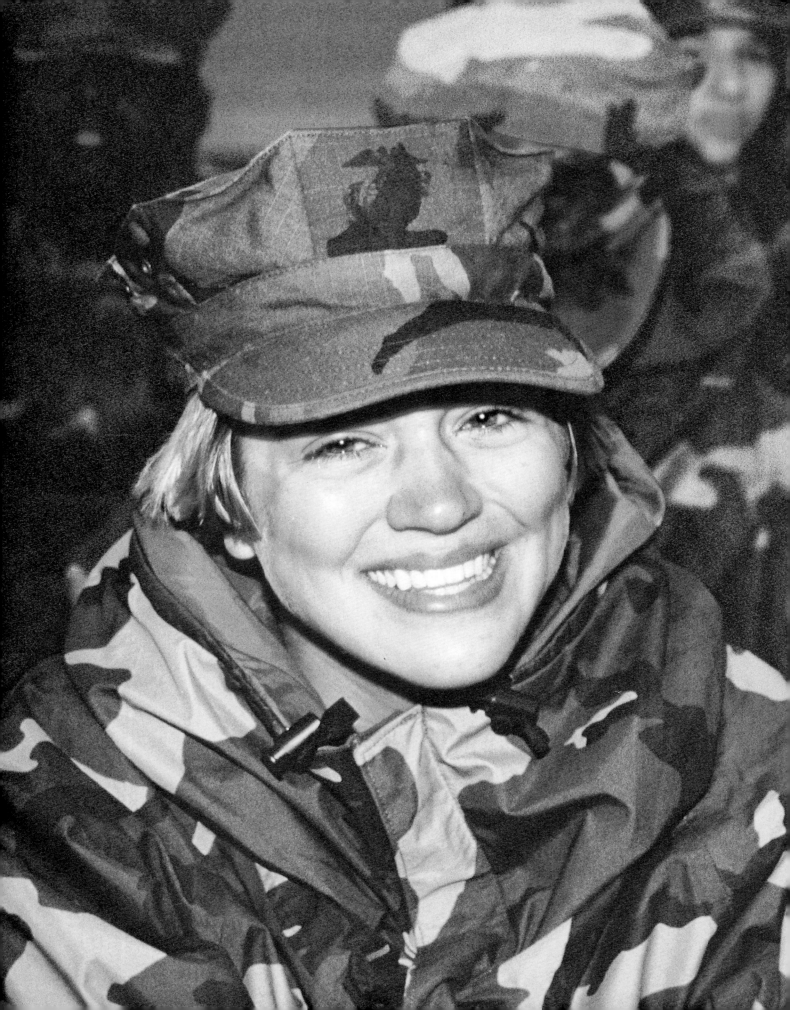

PROGRESSIVE TREADMILL EXERCISE PROGRAM: 30-49 YEARS OF AGE

Week	Activity	Treadmill Speed (mph)	Incline (5%)	Time (min.)	Freq./Wk.	Points/Wk.
1	walk	3.5	flat	20:00	4	7.6
2	walk	4.0	flat	25:00	4	15.9
3	walk	4.0	flat	30:00	4	20.0
4	walk	4.5	flat	25:00	4	22.2
5	walk	4.5	5%	30:00	4	30.2
6	walk/jog	5.0	flat	25:00	4	29.3
7*	walk/jog	5.0	flat	30:00	4	36.0
8	jog	5.5	flat	25:00	4	37.2
9	jog	5.5	5%	25:00	4	41.0
10	jog	6.0	flat	30:00	4	56.0

*By the seventh week, adequate aerobic fitness has been reached (36 aerobic points per week) and it is permissible to continue at this exercise level. By the tenth week, the excellent category has been achieved (56 aerobic points per week). Other combinations of speed, incline, duration and frequency per week can be used to maintain the good or excellent categories of fitness.

JOGGING EXERCISE PROGRAM: 50-59 YEARS OF AGE

Week	Activity	Distance (miles)	Time Goal (min.)	Freq./Wk.	Points/Wk.
1	walk	1.0	18:00	5	5.3
2	walk	2.0	36:00	4	14.7
3	walk	3.0	54:00	3	18.0
4	walk	3.0	52:00	4	25.6
5	walk/jog	2.0	26:00	4	24.9
6	walk/jog	2.0	24:00	4	28.0
7	jog	2.0	22:00	4	31.6
8*	jog	2.0	20:00	4	36.0
9	jog	2.5	27:00	4	41.6
10	jog	2.5	25:00	4	46.0
11	jog	3.0	32:00	4	51.5
12	jog	3.0	30:00	4	56.0

*By the eighth week, a minimum aerobic fitness level has been reached (36 aerobic points per week) but it is suggested that a higher level of fitness be achieved. By the twelfth week of the program, a total of 56 points per week is being earned, consistent with the excellent category of aerobic fitness.

PROGRESSIVE TREADMILL EXERCISE PROGRAM: 50 YEARS OF AGE AND OLDER

Week	Activity	Treadmill Speed (mph)	Incline (%)	Time (min.)	Freq./Wk.	Points/Wk.
1	walk	3.0	flat	20:00	4	4.0
2	walk	3.0	flat	25:00	4	6.0
3	walk	3.0	flat	30:00	4	8.0
4	walk	3.5	flat	25:00	4	10.5
5	walk	3.5	flat	30:00	4	13.5
6	walk	3.75	flat	25:00	4	13.2
7	walk	3.75	flat	30:00	5	20.7
8	walk	4.0	flat	30:00	5	25.0
9*	walk	4.0	flat	45:00	5	40.0
10*	walk	4.0	5%	45:00	4	35.2

*Either 4.0 mph at no incline for 45:00 minutes, 5 times per week, or 45:00 minutes with a 5% incline, 4 times per week, can be used to achieve adequate fitness. Both training programs will produce the good category of aerobic fitness. For individuals over age 60, fast walking or slow jogging on a treadmill is discouraged unless the subject has been exercising regularly before age 60. In such cases, continued treadmill exercise is permissible past age 60.

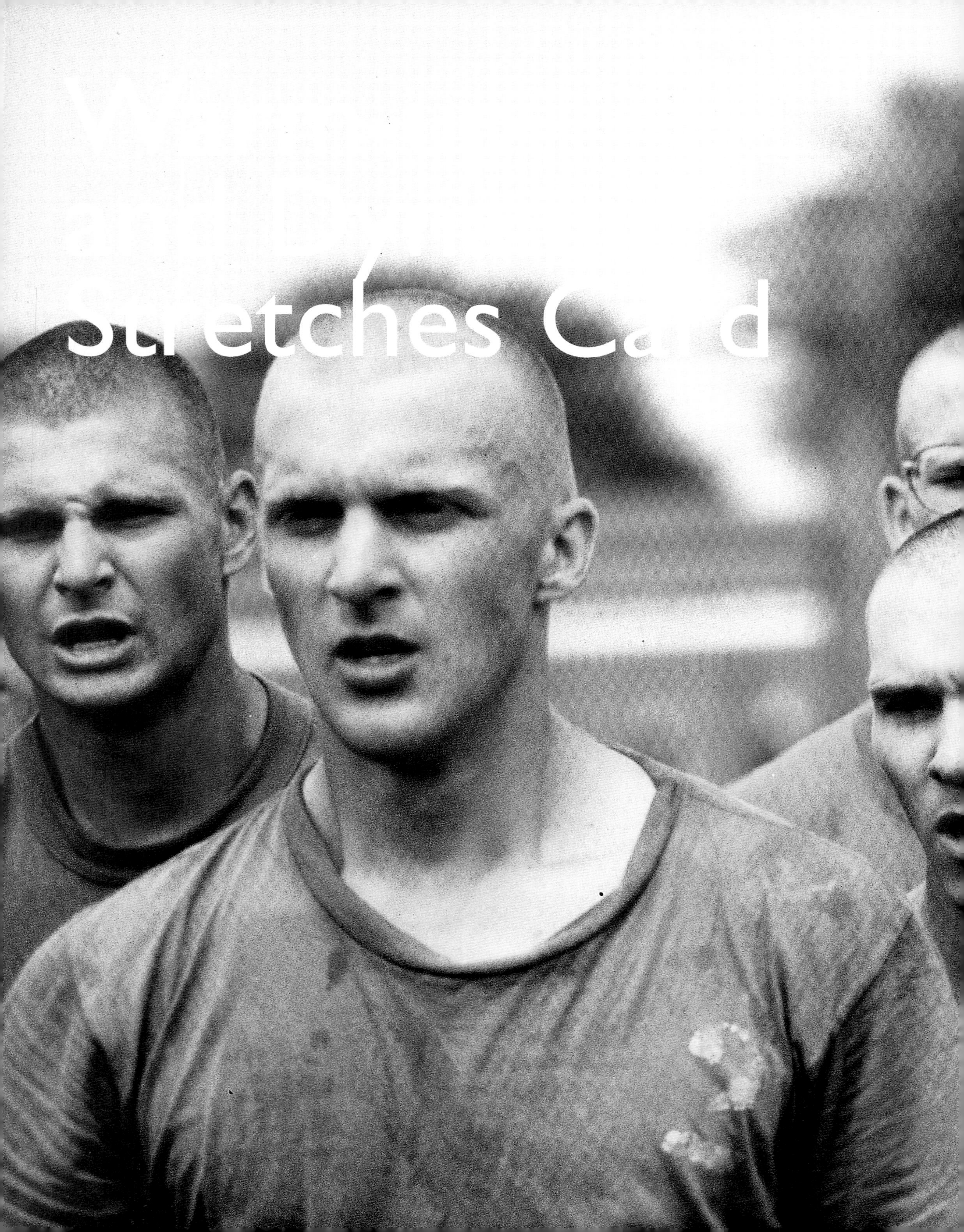
Stretches Card

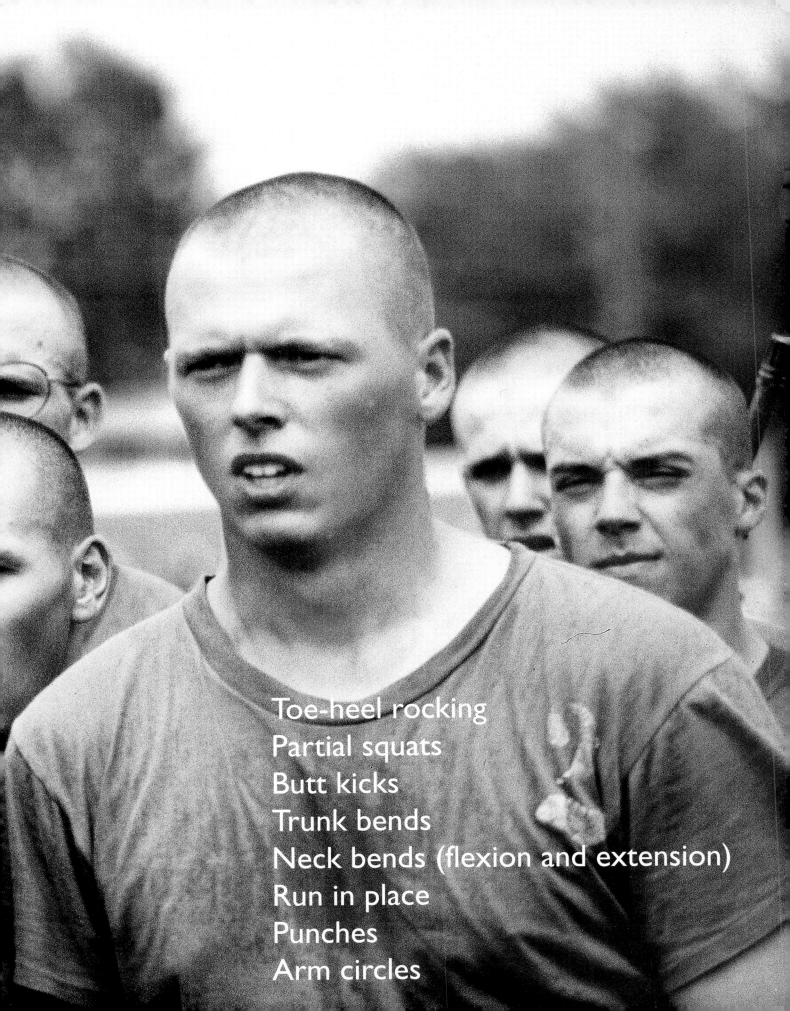

Toe-heel rocking
Partial squats
Butt kicks
Trunk bends
Neck bends (flexion and extension)
Run in place
Punches
Arm circles

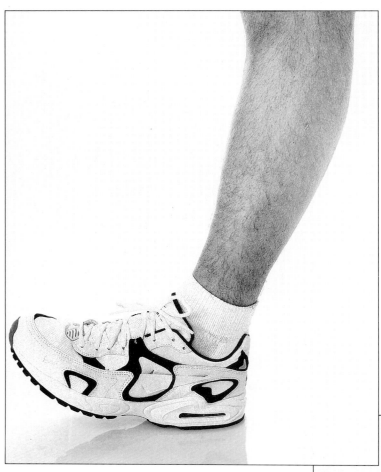

1. Toe-heel rocking

Rock back onto the heels then forward onto the toes. Repeat 10 to 15 times.

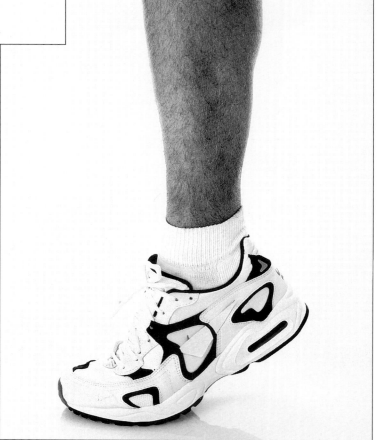

PLANTAR FASCIITIS

The plantar fascia is a thick fibrous material on the bottom of the foot. It is attached to the heel bone (calcaneus), fans forward toward the toes, and acts like a bowstring to maintain the arch of the foot.

A problem may occur when part of this inflexible fascia is repeatedly placed under tension, as in running. Tension causes an overload that produces an inflammation usually at the point where the fascia is attached to the heel bone. The result is pain.

Plantar fascia injury may also occur at midsole or near the toes. Since it is difficult to rest the foot, the problem gradually becomes worse because the condition is aggravated with every step. In severe cases, the heel is visibly swollen. The problem may progress rapidly;

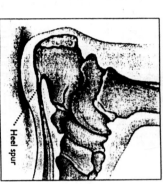

Heel spur

shoes, and sedentary activities all help the injury to mend. You should return to full activity gradually.

Rest. Use pain as your guide. If your foot is too painful, rest it.

Ice. Ice the sore area for 30 to 60 minutes several times a day to reduce the inflammation. Apply a plastic bag of crushed ice over a towel (or a bag of

ed. Your doctor will tell you where you can get heel pads; they are available at some medical supply and sporting goods stores.

Shoes. Poorly fitting shoes can cause plantar fasciitis. The best type of shoe to wear is a good running shoe with excellent support. You should choose the one that fits best. Experiment with your athletic shoes to find a pair that is comfortable and causes fewer symptoms.

Orthoses. Orthoses (sometimes misnamed "orthotics") are shoe inserts that your doctor will prescribe if necessary.

Taping. Your doctor may tape your foot to maintain the arch; this will take some of the ten-

vate the problem. The injury may be precipitated by sudden weight increase, changes in activity level, or sudden return to activity after a long period of rest (e.g., after being in a cast). To maintain cardiovascular fitness, weight-bearing sports can be temporarily replaced by non-weight-bearing sports (e.g., swimming, cycling). Weight training can be used to maintain leg strength.

When recovering from plantar fasciitis, return to sports activities slowly. If you have a lot of pain either during the activity or the following morning, you are doing too much.

Using heel pads or changing to different or new shoes may help the problem.

EXERCISES

PLANTAR FASCIITIS

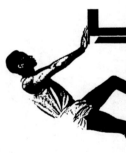

Tibia

Fibula

Heel bone (calcaneus)

Inflamed fascia.

Exercises

Shin Curls. Run your injured foot slowly up and down the shin of your other leg as you try to grab the shin with your toes. A similar exercise can be done curling your toes around a tin can.

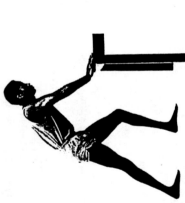

Stretching

Repeat _____ Times _____ times/day

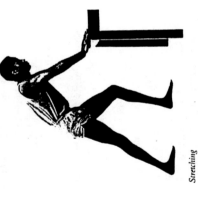

Shin Curls

Repeat _____ Times _____ times/day

Stretches. Stand at arm's length

your back knee locked and your front knee bent. Slowly lean toward the table, pressing forward until a moderate stretch is felt in the calf muscles of your straight leg. Hold 15 seconds. Keeping both heels on the floor, bend the knee of your straight leg until a moderate stretch is felt in your Achilles tendon. (Tendons attach muscles to bones; the Achilles tendon attaches the muscles of the calf to the heel bone.) Hold 15 seconds more. You should feel a moderate pull in your muscles and tendon, but no pain. Change legs and stretch the other leg.

➤ THE INJURY

Plantar fasciitis (heel-spur syndrome) is a common problem among people who are active in sports, particularly runners.

It starts as a dull intermittent pain in the heel which may progress to a sharp persistent pain. Classically, it is worse in the morning with the first few steps, after sitting, after standing or walking, and at the beginning of sporting activity.

034/w209-29-55 0   VN# 3069
MARSH, SUSAN ELIZABETH   ABS
F 51 12/08/1951   310-670-1046
07/17/03   ISCCF   ANITA YVONNE
DMPG: AGZARIAN,   2   PR 07/17/03
w209-29-55 3069

PRESENTED AS AN EDUCATIONAL SERVICE BY SYNTEX LABORATORIES, INC.

The inflammatory reaction of the heel bone may produce spike-like projections of new bone called heel spurs. They sometimes show on x-rays. They do not cause the initial pain, nor do they cause the initial problem: they are a result of the problem. But later, having to walk on spurs may cause sharp pain.

Contributing Factors

- *Flat (pronated) feet*
- *High arched, rigid feet*
- *Poor shoe support*
- *Toe running, hill running*
- *Soft terrain (e.g., running on sand)*
- *Increasing age*
- *Sudden weight increase*
- *Sudden increase in activity level*
- *Family tendency*

Treatment

Improvement may take longer than expected, especially if the condition has existed for a long time. During recovery, loss of excess weight, good utes after activity:

Medication. If your condition developed recently, anti-inflammatory/analgesic medication, coupled with heel pads (see below), may be all that is necessary to relieve pain and reduce inflammation. If no pain relief has occurred after 2 or 3 weeks, however, your doctor may inject either cortisone or local anesthetic directly into the tender area.

Physical Therapy. The initial objective of physical therapy (when needed) is to decrease the inflammation. Later, the small muscles of the foot can be strengthened to support the weakened plantar fascia.

Heel Pads. A heel pad of felt, sponge, or a newer synthetic material can help to spread, equalize, and absorb the shock as your heel lands, thus easing the pressure on the plantar fascia. It may be necessary to cut a hole in the heel pad so the painful area will not be irritat- the following exercises are designed to strengthen the small muscles of the foot to help support the damaged area. If done regularly, they will help prevent reinjury. DO EACH PRESCRIBED EXERCISE TWO TIMES A DAY OR AS OFTEN AS YOUR DOCTOR RECOMMENDS.

Surgery. Surgery is rarely required for plantar fasciitis. It would be considered only if all forms of more conservative treatment fail and if the pain is still incapacitating after several months of treatment. When needed, surgery involves removal of the bone spur and release of the plantar fascia.

SPORTS

Plantar fasciitis can be aggravated by all weight-bearing sports. Any sport where the foot lands repeatedly, such as running or jogging, can aggra-

Towel Curls. Place towel on the floor and curl it toward you, using only the toes of your injured foot. Resistance can be increased with a weight on the end of the towel. Relax, then repeat the towel curl.

Exercises

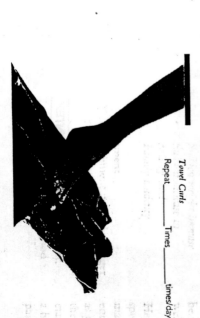

Towel Curls
Repeat _____ Times _____ times/day

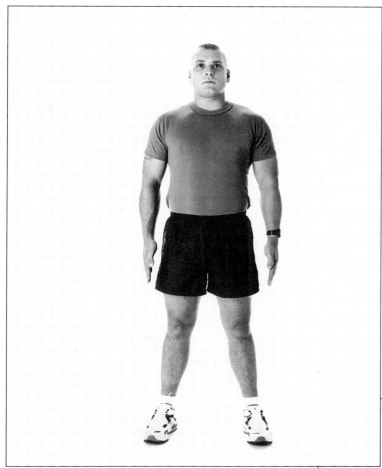

2. Partial squats
Stand with feet shoulder-width apart, arms at the sides.

Keeping heels on the deck, partially squat until hands are near mid-calf. The knees should bend only to about 60 degrees. Repeat 10 to 15 times.

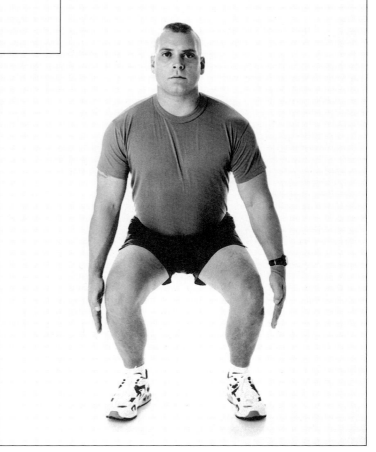

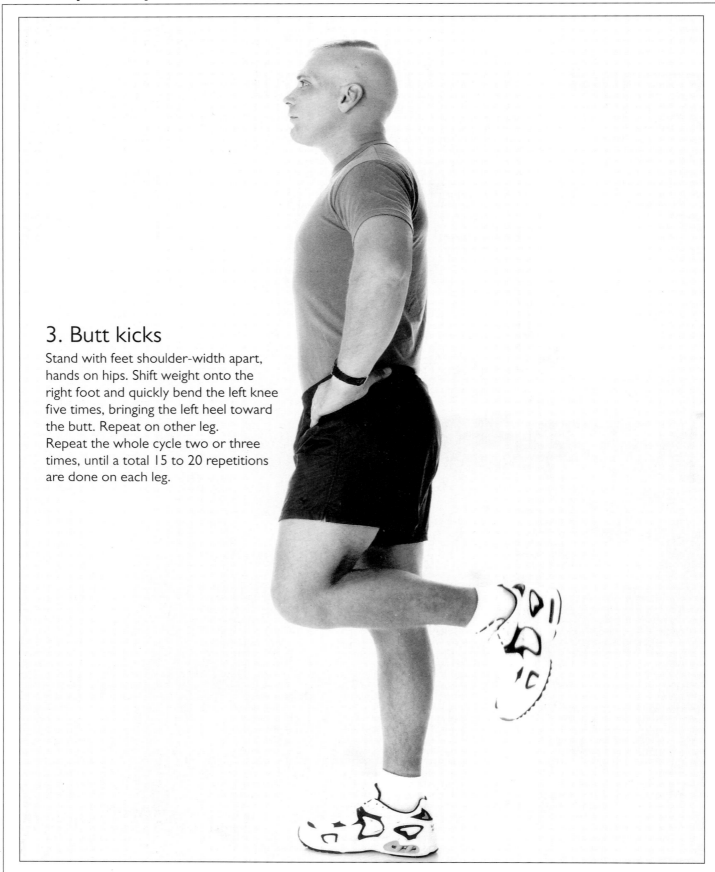

3. Butt kicks

Stand with feet shoulder-width apart, hands on hips. Shift weight onto the right foot and quickly bend the left knee five times, bringing the left heel toward the butt. Repeat on other leg. Repeat the whole cycle two or three times, until a total 15 to 20 repetitions are done on each leg.

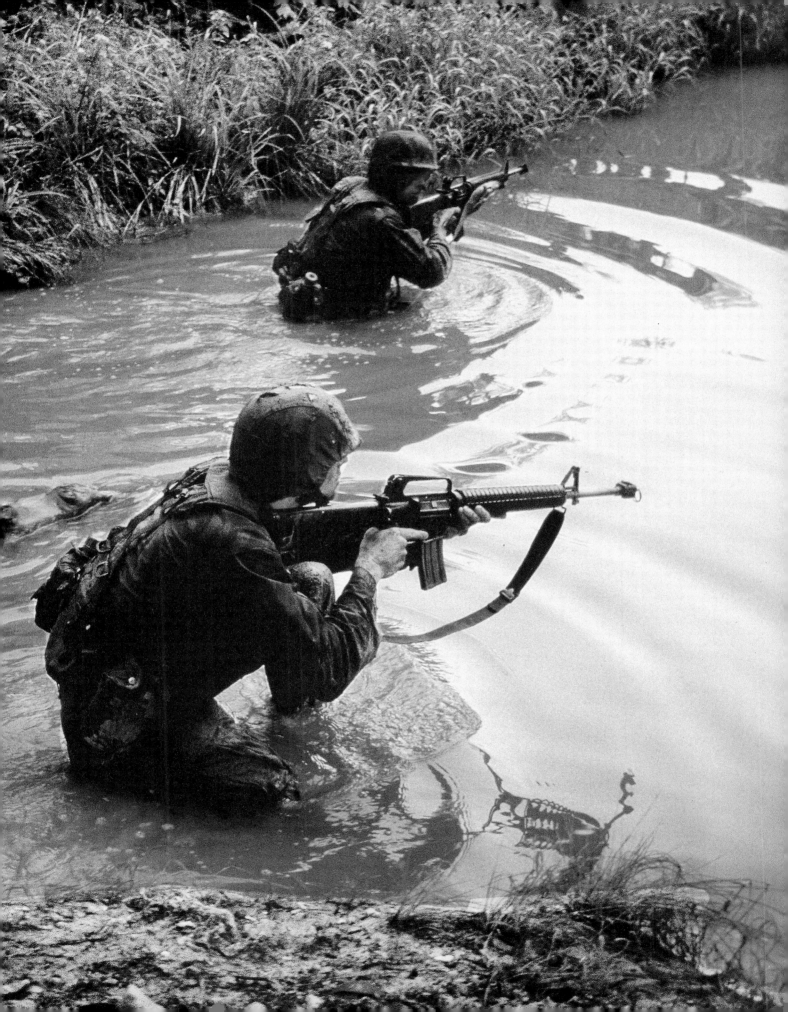

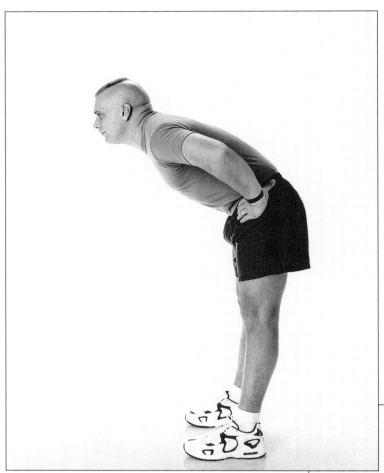

4. Trunk bends

Trunk bend (front to back)

Flex the trunk forward to a 45 degree angle.
Then slightly hyperextend the trunk backward.
Five to 10 repetitions.

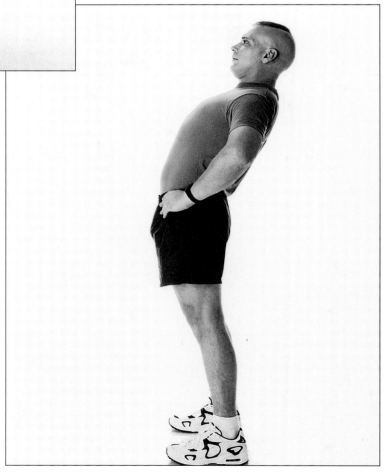

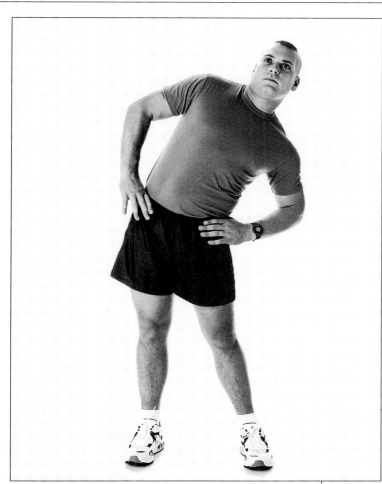

Trunk bend (side to side)
Bend the trunk to the left side,
then to the right side.
Five to 10 repetitions.

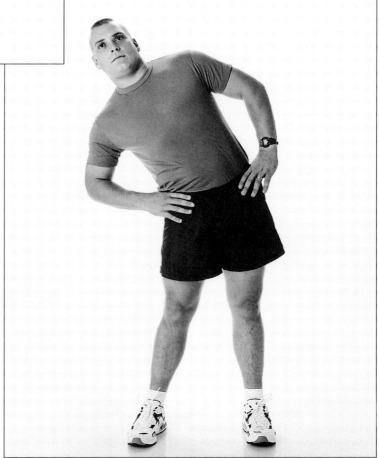

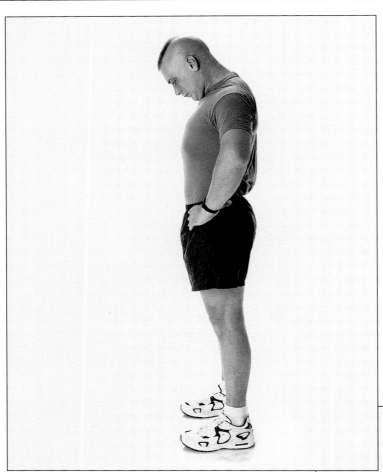

5. Neck bends
Neck bend (front to back)
Flex the neck forward, bringing the chin toward the chest. Extend the head back. Five to 10 repetitions.

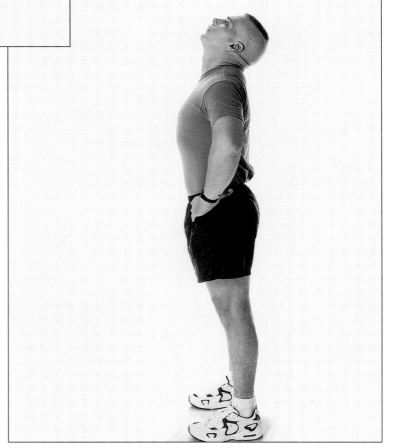

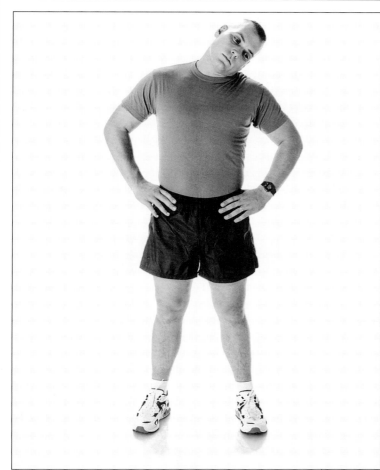

Neck bend (side to side)

Tilt the head to the left side, bringing the left ear toward the left shoulder. Repeat to the right side. Five to 10 repetitions.

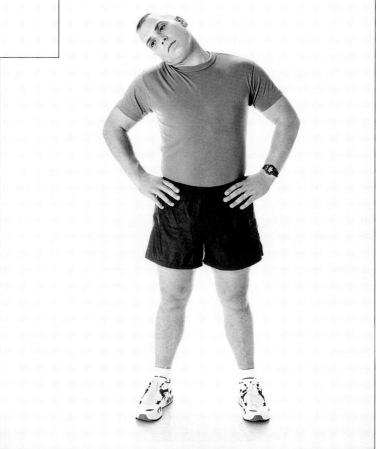

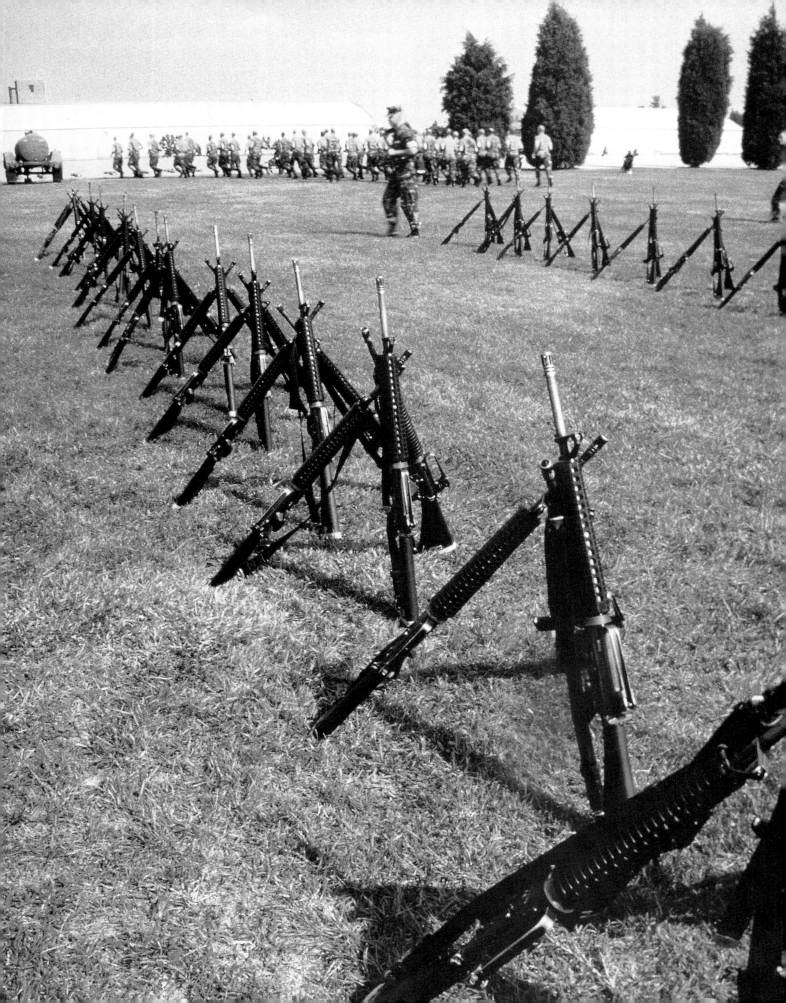

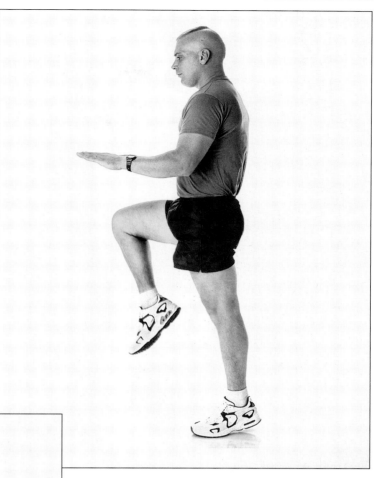

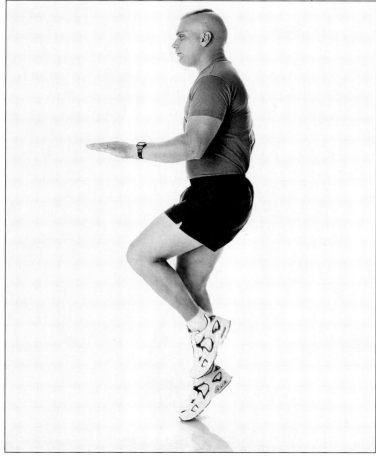

6. Run in place: "Double-time"

Raise knees to hands, and hold at waist level and parallel to the ground. Keep knee as high as possible. Keep back at right angle to deck. Do not tilt torso front or back. Begin slowly and gradually increase tempo to 180 steps per minute.

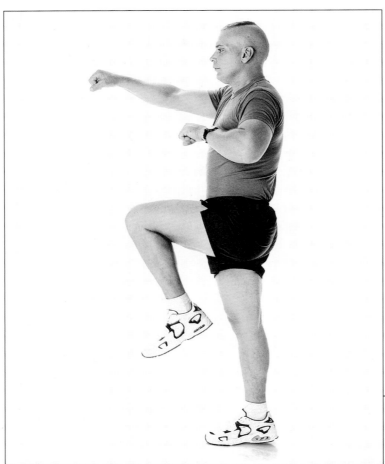

7. Punches

Throw easy punches to the front of the body, while double-time stepping. Keep punches parallel to the ground. Five to 10 repetitions.

Throw easy punches straight up to the sky. Five to 10 repetitions.

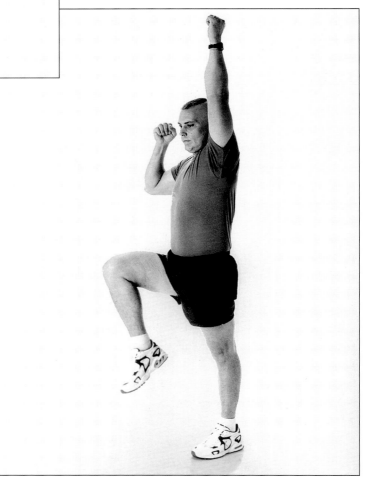

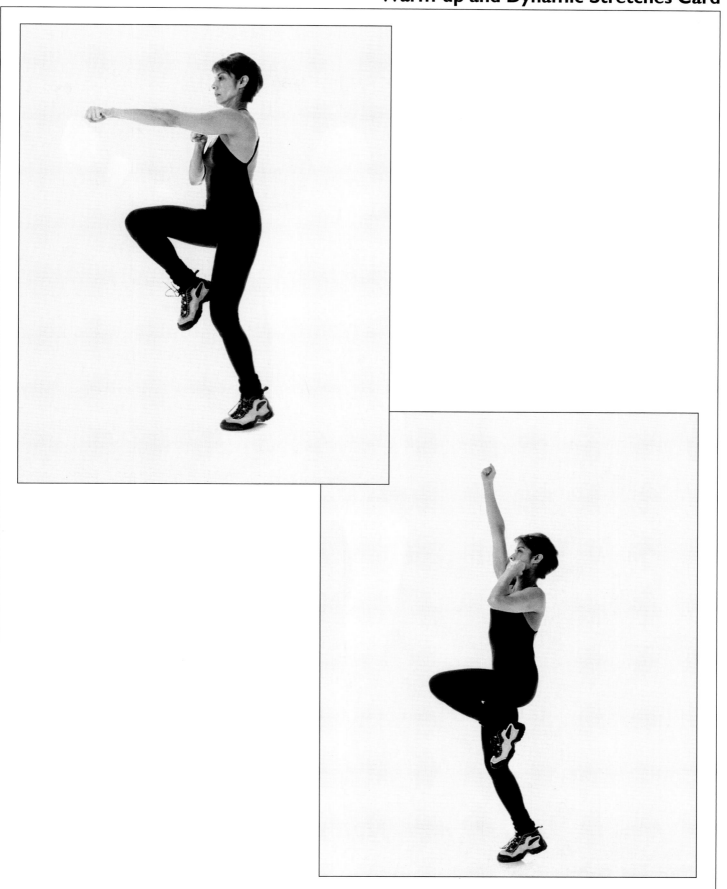

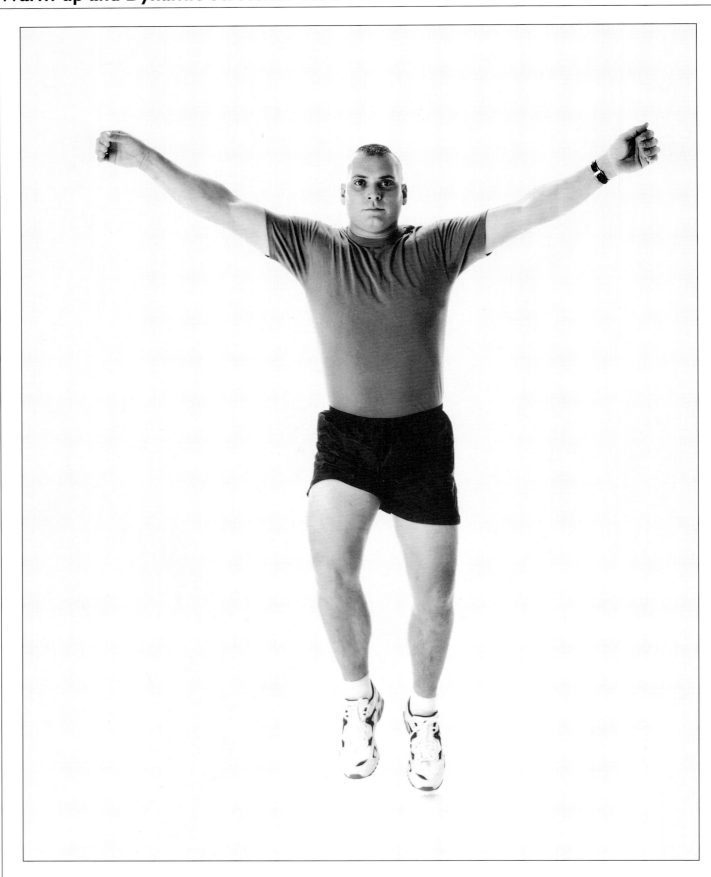

8. Arm circles while double-time stepping

Begin small, then enlarge the diameter of the arm circles.
Repeat in other direction. Five to 10 repetitions.

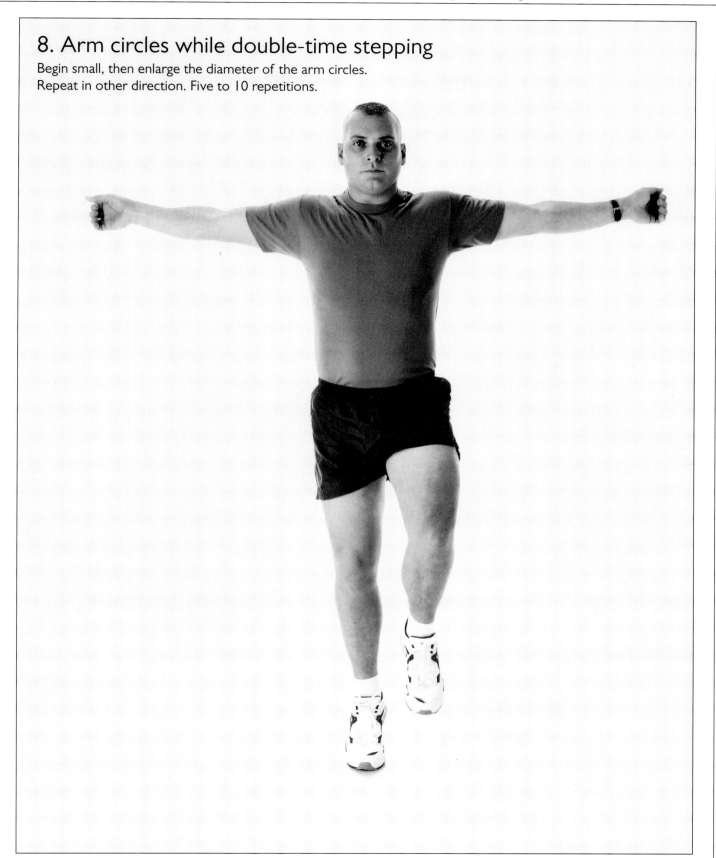

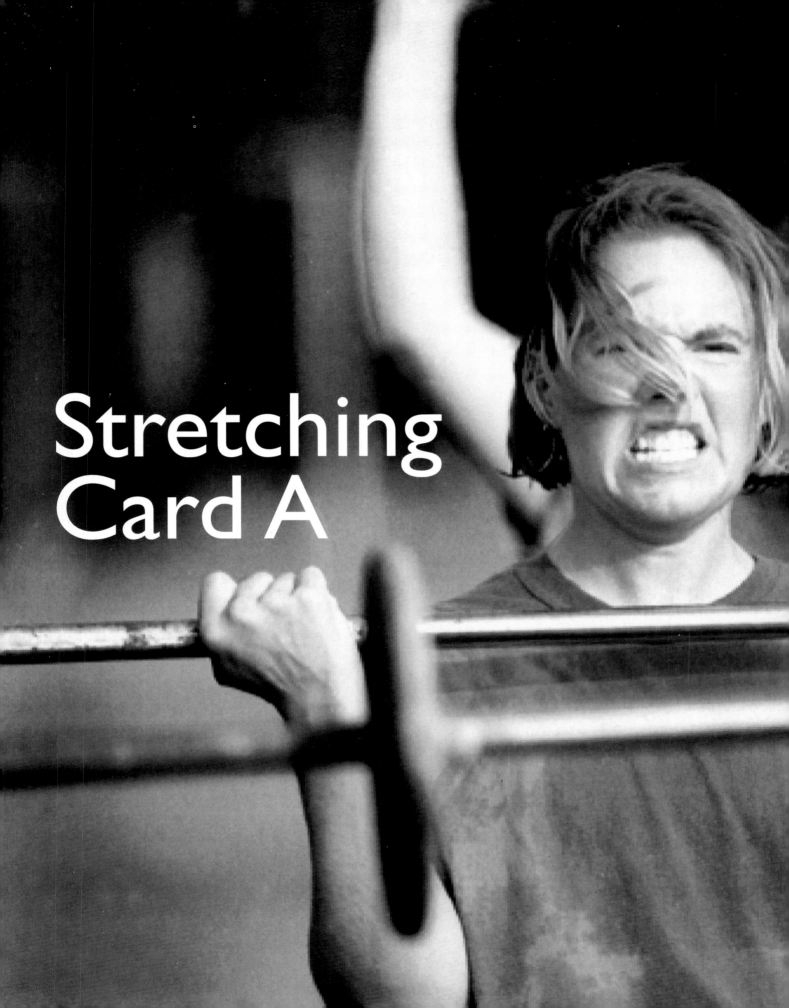

Stretching
Card A

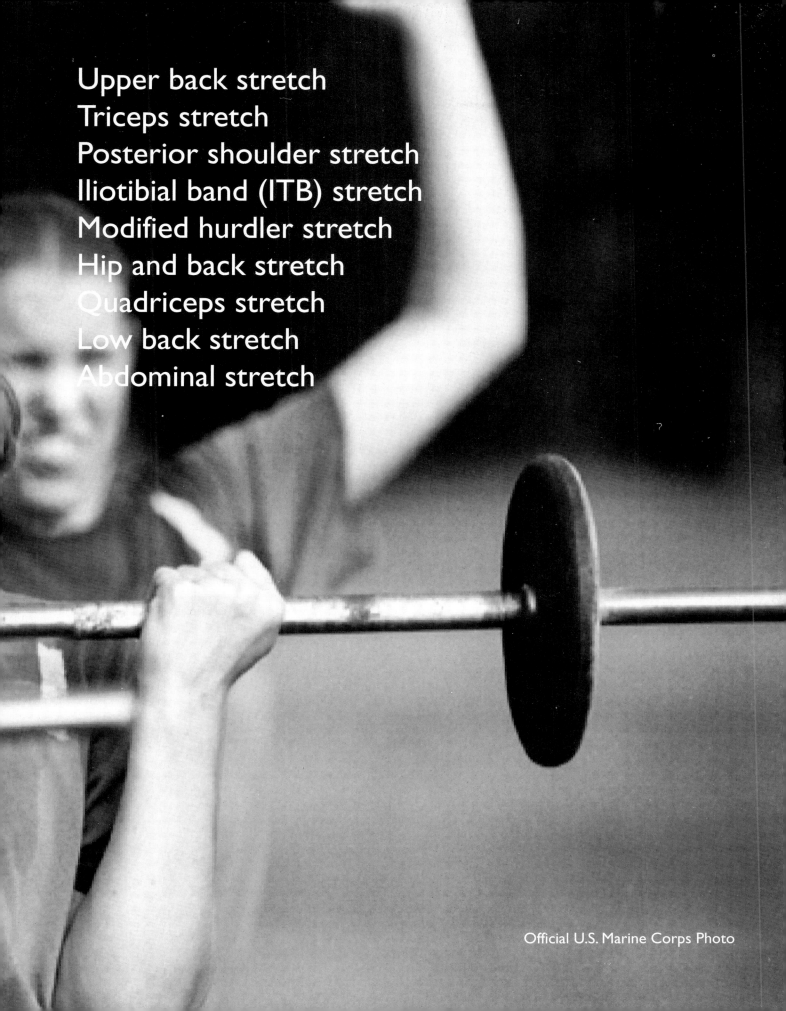

Upper back stretch
Triceps stretch
Posterior shoulder stretch
Iliotibial band (ITB) stretch
Modified hurdler stretch
Hip and back stretch
Quadriceps stretch
Low back stretch
Abdominal stretch

1. Upper back stretch

Extend the arms and clasp the hands in front of the chest. Push the arms forward, rounding the shoulders and upper back. The stretch should be felt over the upper back. This stretches the lower trapezius and posterior deltoid muscles of the upper back.

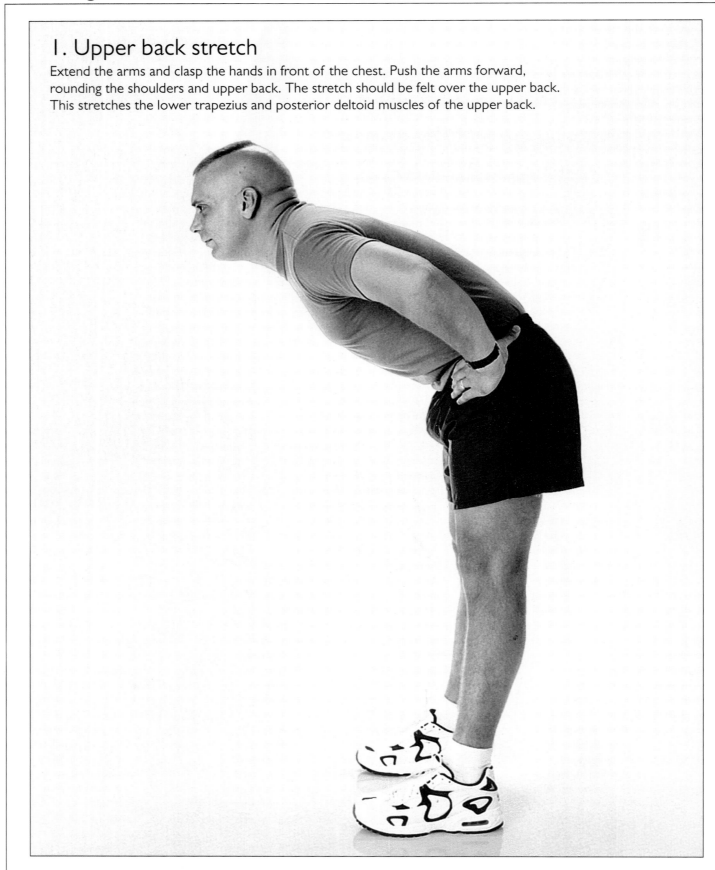

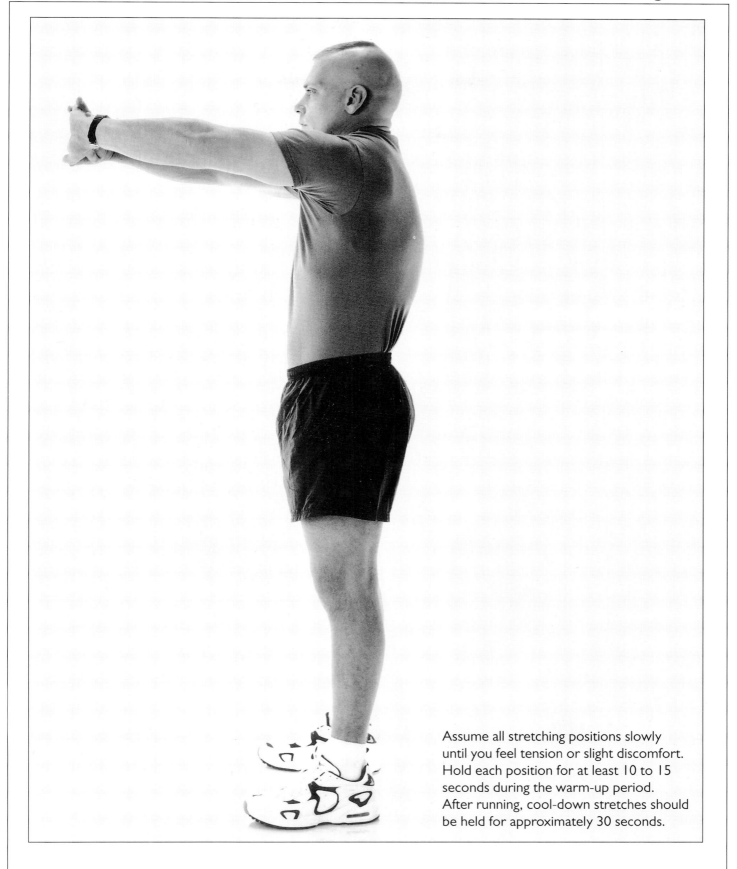

Assume all stretching positions slowly until you feel tension or slight discomfort. Hold each position for at least 10 to 15 seconds during the warm-up period. After running, cool-down stretches should be held for approximately 30 seconds.

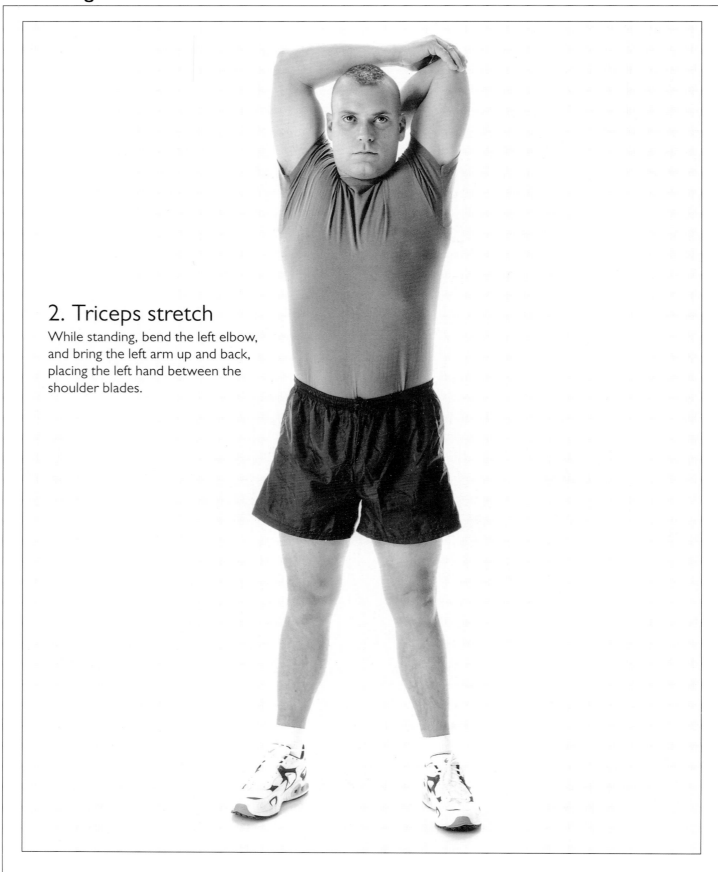

2. Triceps stretch

While standing, bend the left elbow, and bring the left arm up and back, placing the left hand between the shoulder blades.

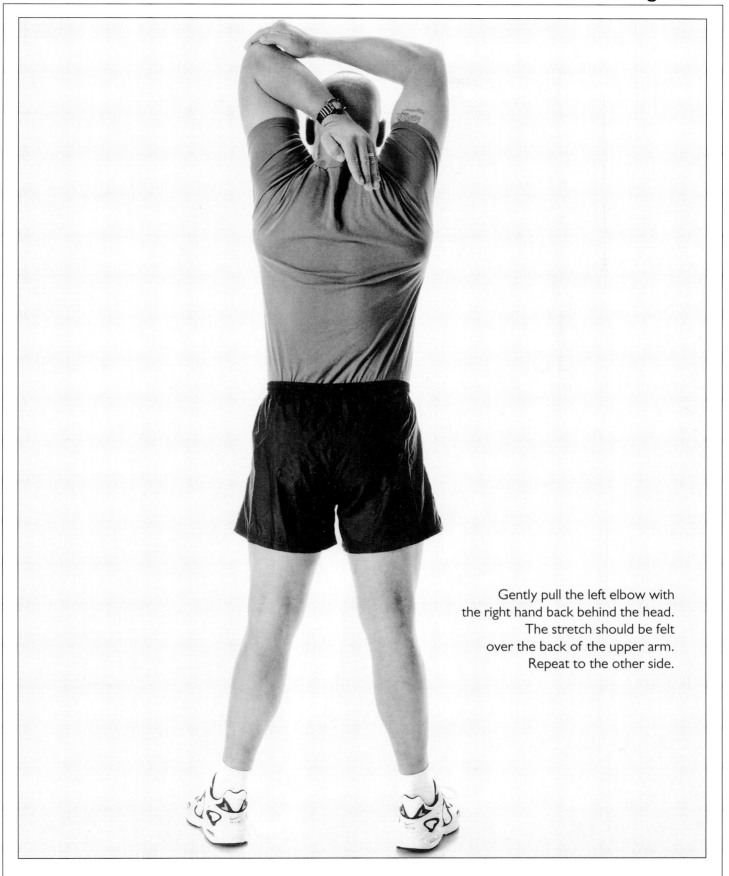

Gently pull the left elbow with
the right hand back behind the head.
The stretch should be felt
over the back of the upper arm.
Repeat to the other side.

3. Posterior shoulder stretch

Bend the left elbow, and bring the
left arm across the chest. Give a gentle
pull over the posterior left shoulder.
Repeat to the other side.

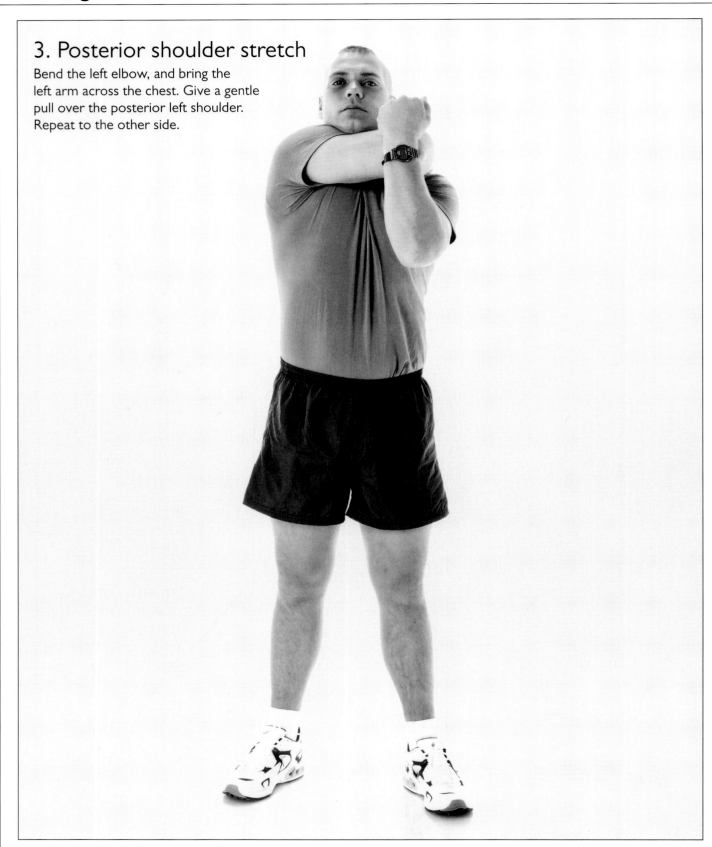

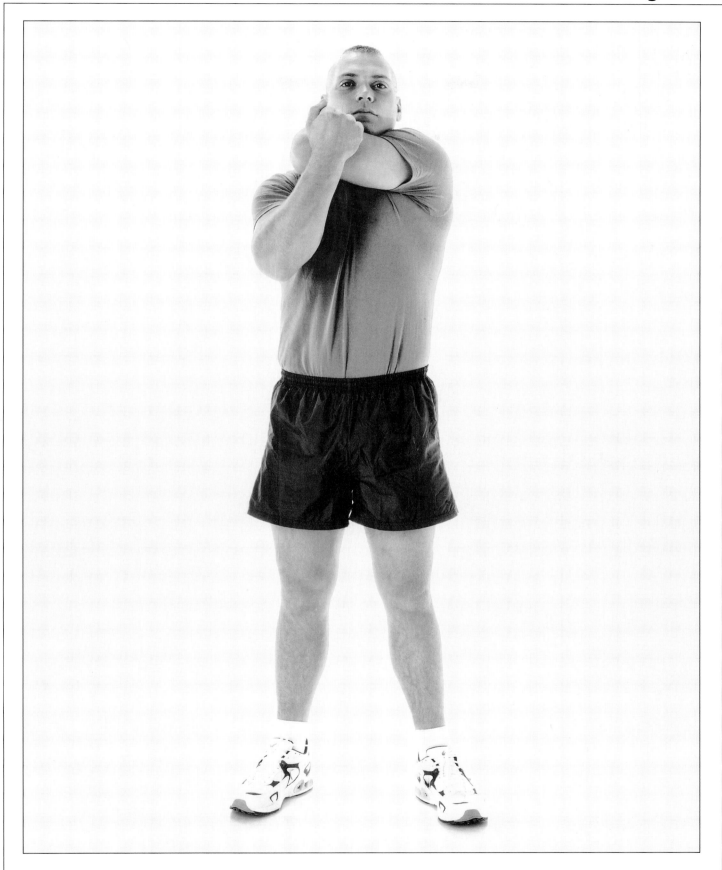

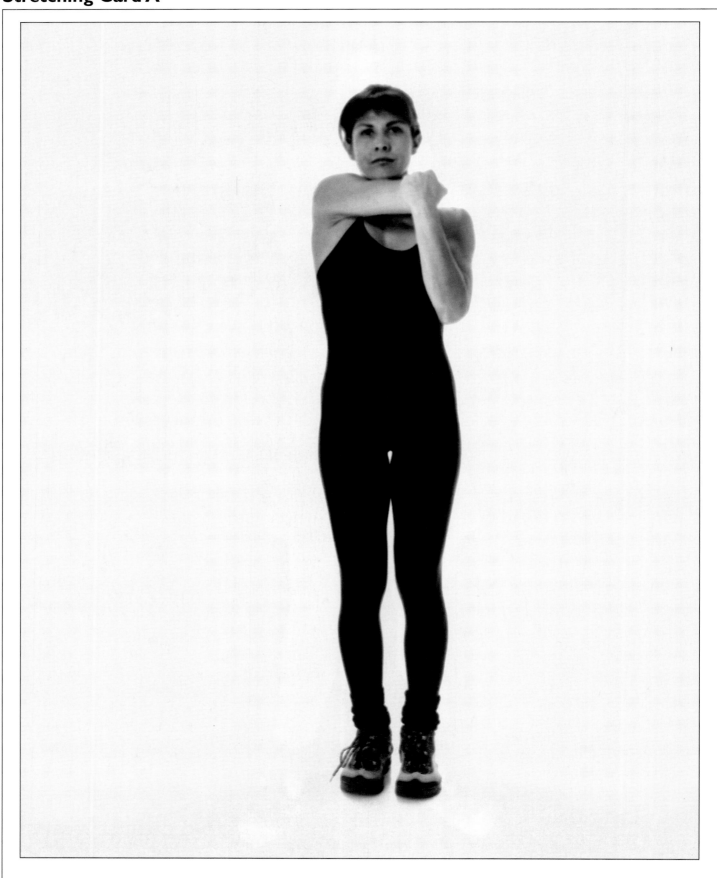

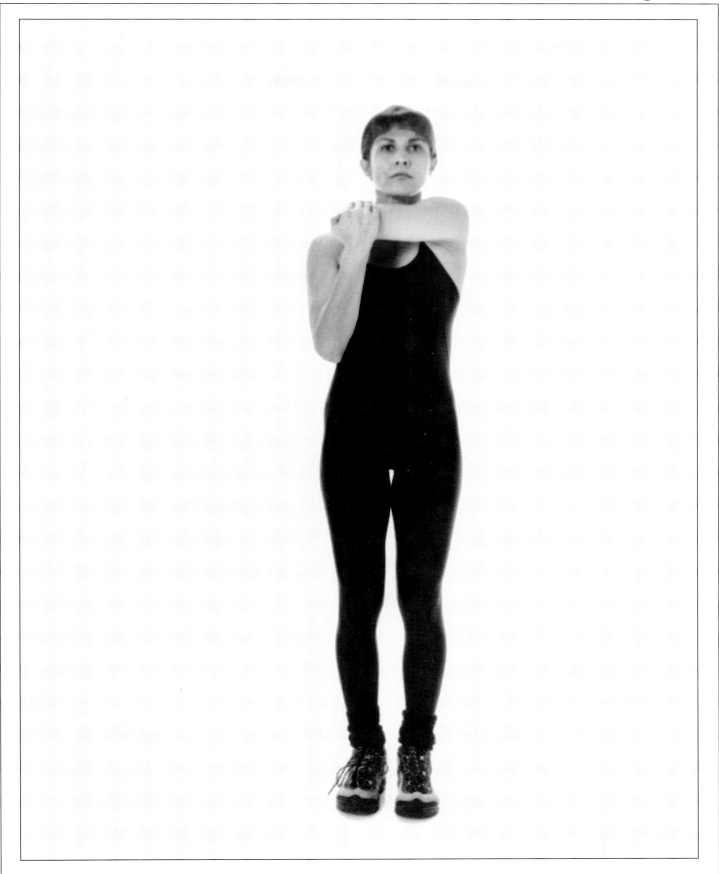

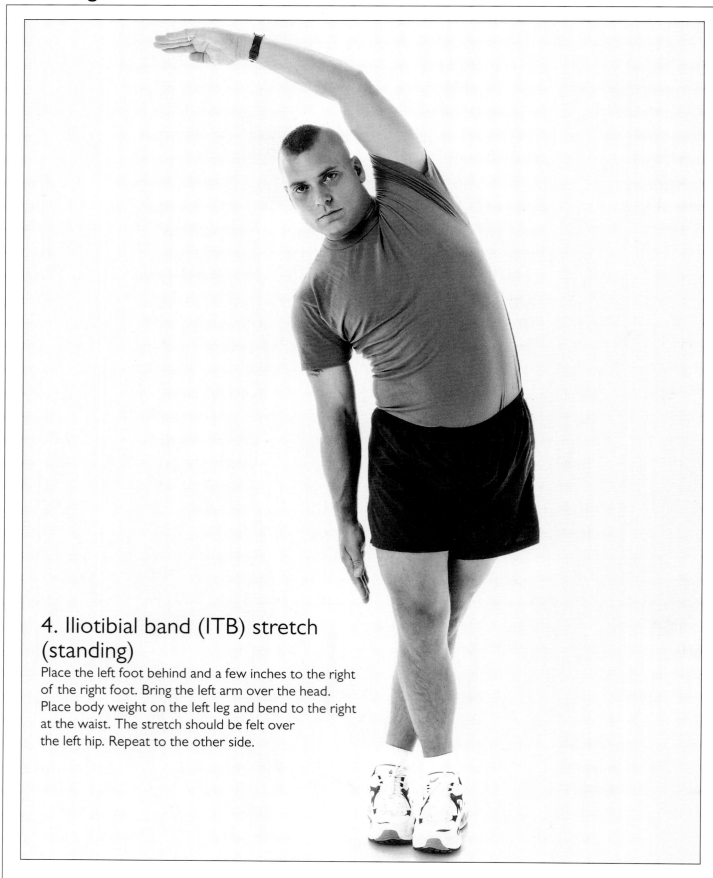

4. Iliotibial band (ITB) stretch (standing)

Place the left foot behind and a few inches to the right of the right foot. Bring the left arm over the head. Place body weight on the left leg and bend to the right at the waist. The stretch should be felt over the left hip. Repeat to the other side.

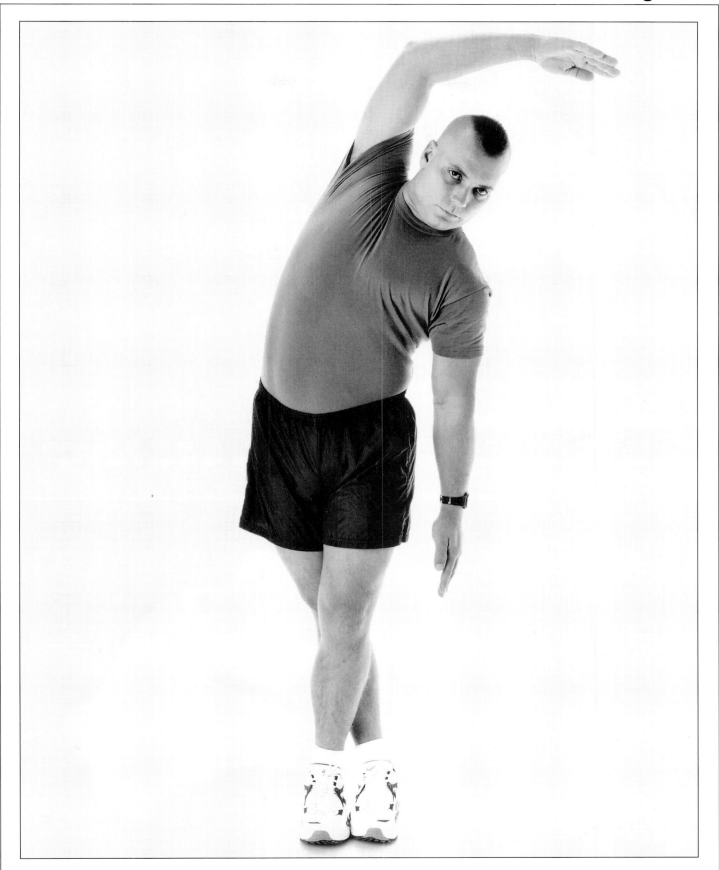

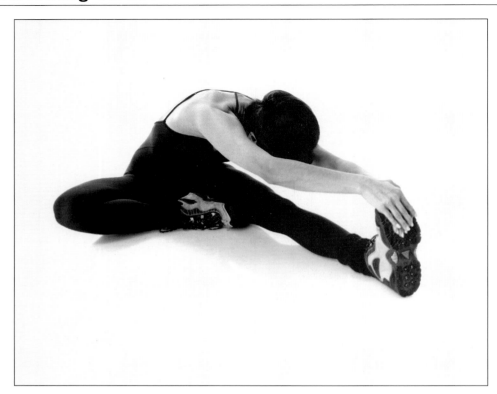

5. Modified hurdler stretch

From a sitting position, extend the left leg out while tucking the right leg in front of the hips with the knee pointing outward. Bend the torso forward toward the left knee. The stretch should be felt over the back of the left thigh. Repeat to the other side.

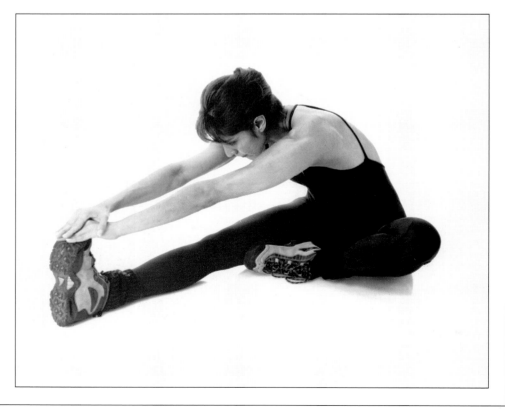

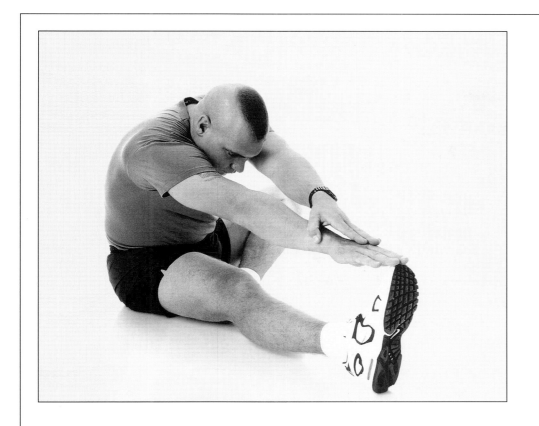

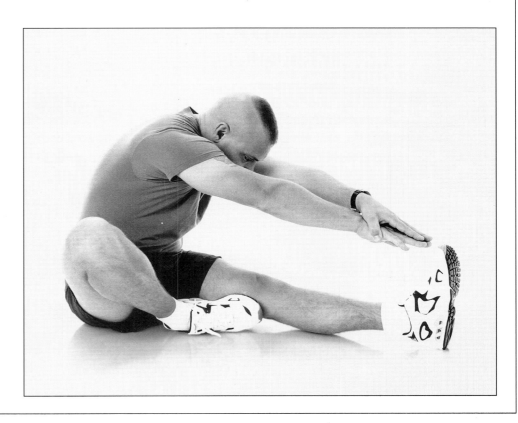

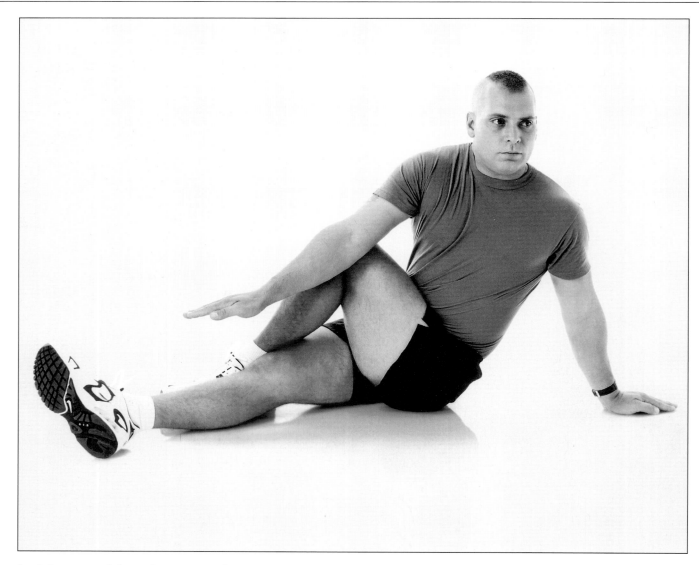

6. Hip and back stretch

Sit on the deck with the right leg extended straight and the left leg crossed over the right leg by bending the left knee and placing the left foot on the deck next to the right knee. Turn the upper torso to the left, pushing the left knee to the right with the right elbow. The stretch should be felt over the lower back and the left hip. Repeat to the other side.

7. Quadriceps stretch

Lying on the left side, bend the left hip and knee to 90 degrees. Grasp the right ankle with the right hand and pull the right knee straight back. Do not hyperextend the low back. The stretch should be felt over the front of the right thigh. Repeat to the other side.

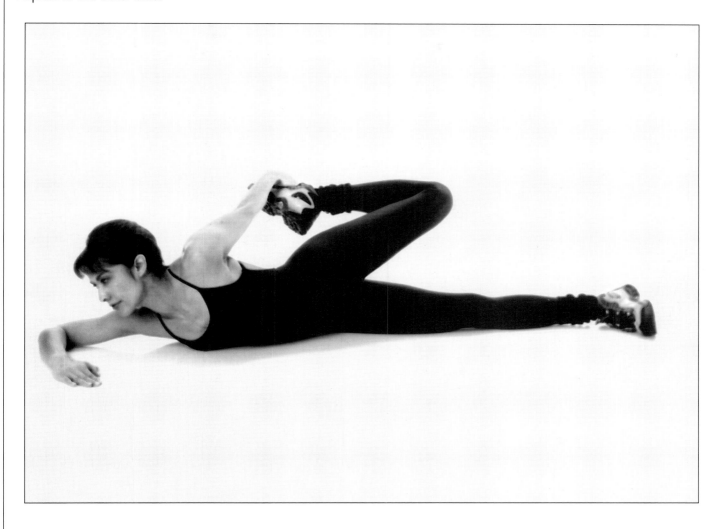

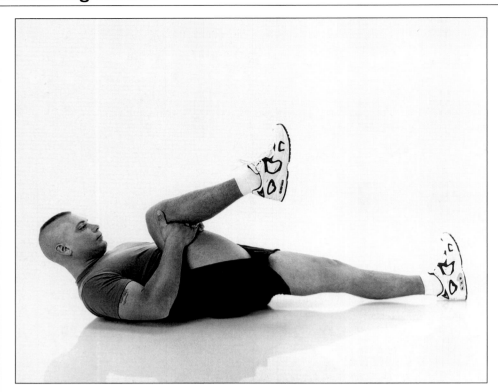

8. Low back stretch

Lying with the back flat against the deck, bring the right knee toward the chest, grasping the right knee. Gently pull the knee tight into the chest. The left leg should remain on the deck. The stretch should be felt along the lower back to the right buttock. Repeat to the other side.

NOTE: It is important in this exercise to grab under the thigh rather than the knee.

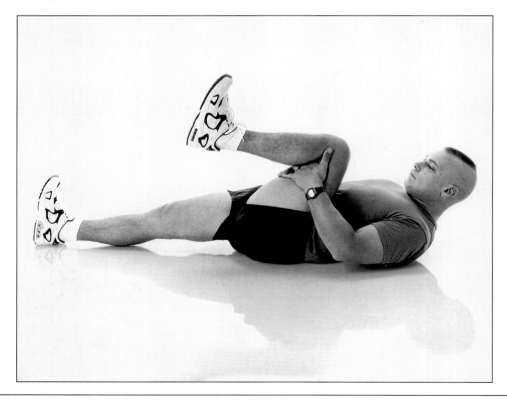

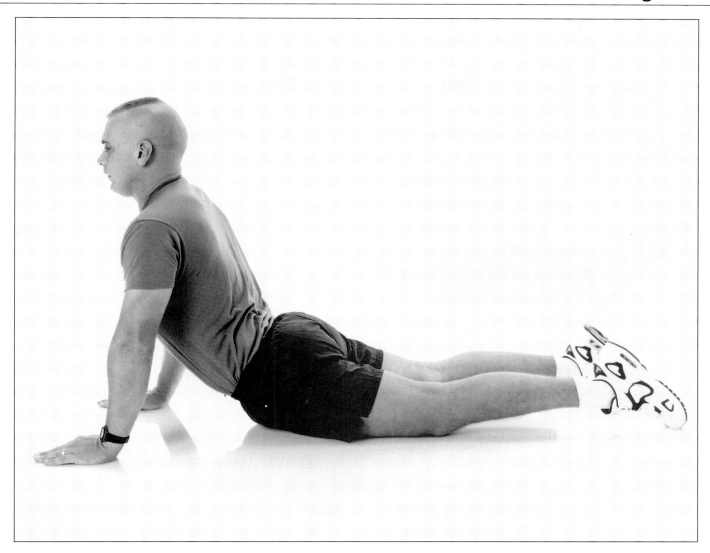

9. Abdominal stretch

Lie on the stomach with the hands placed near the shoulders as in the down position of a pushup. Slowly raise the upper body up, keeping the waist on the deck. The stretch should be felt over the abdomen and works out the abdominals, obliques, latissimus dorsi, and biceps.

Stretching Card B

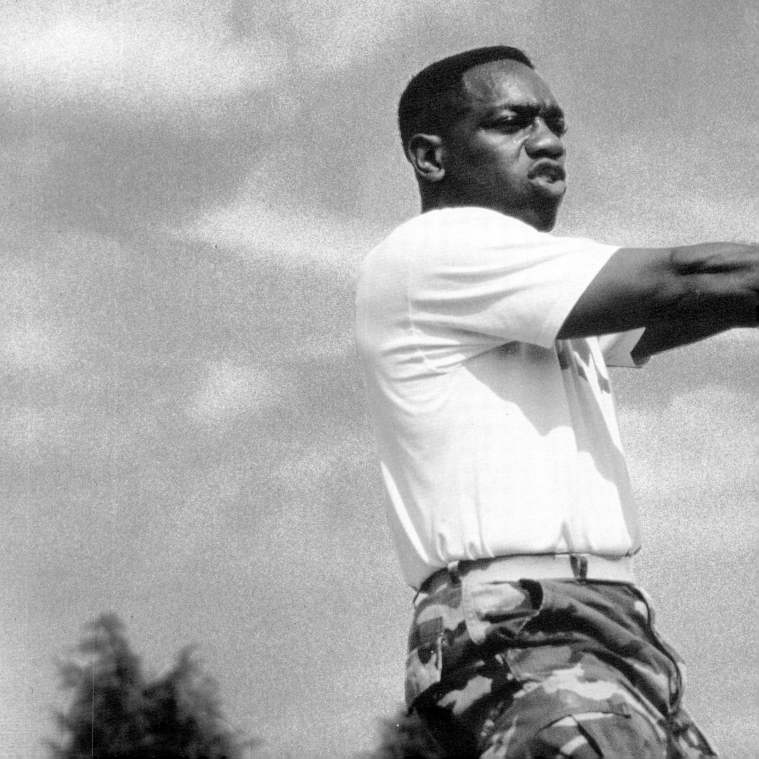

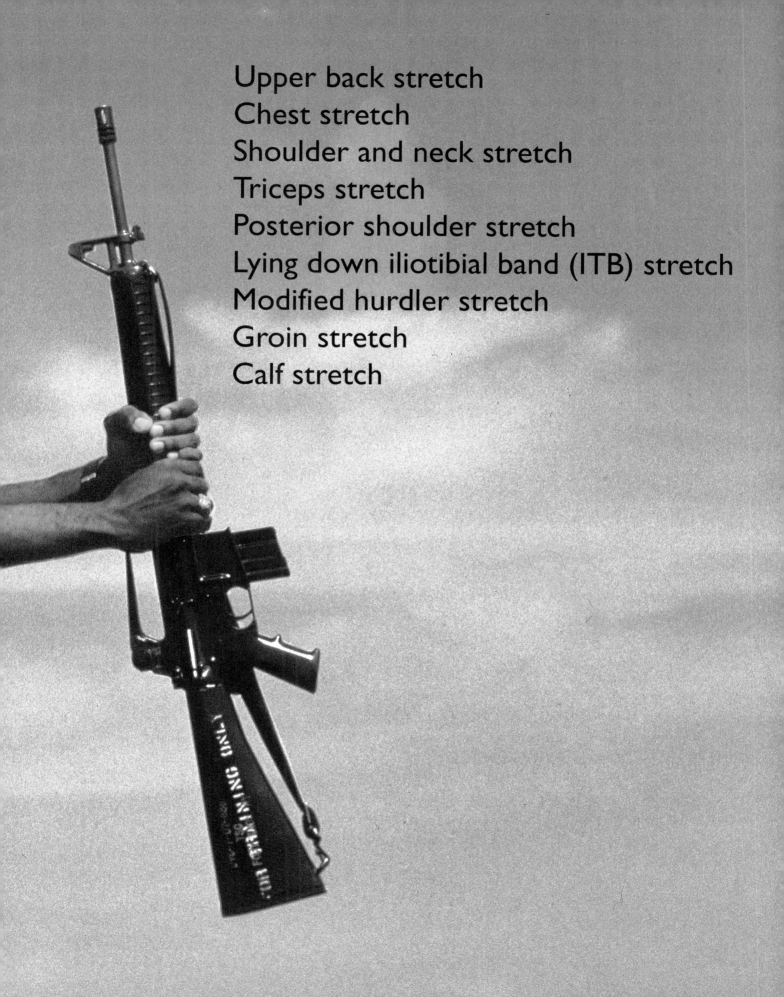

Upper back stretch
Chest stretch
Shoulder and neck stretch
Triceps stretch
Posterior shoulder stretch
Lying down iliotibial band (ITB) stretch
Modified hurdler stretch
Groin stretch
Calf stretch

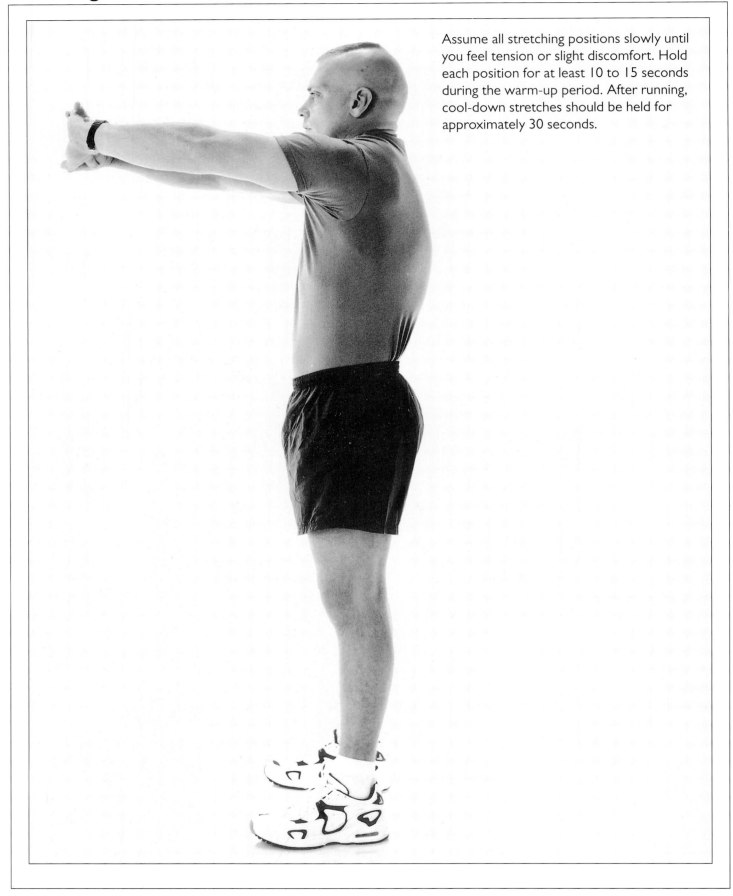

Assume all stretching positions slowly until you feel tension or slight discomfort. Hold each position for at least 10 to 15 seconds during the warm-up period. After running, cool-down stretches should be held for approximately 30 seconds.

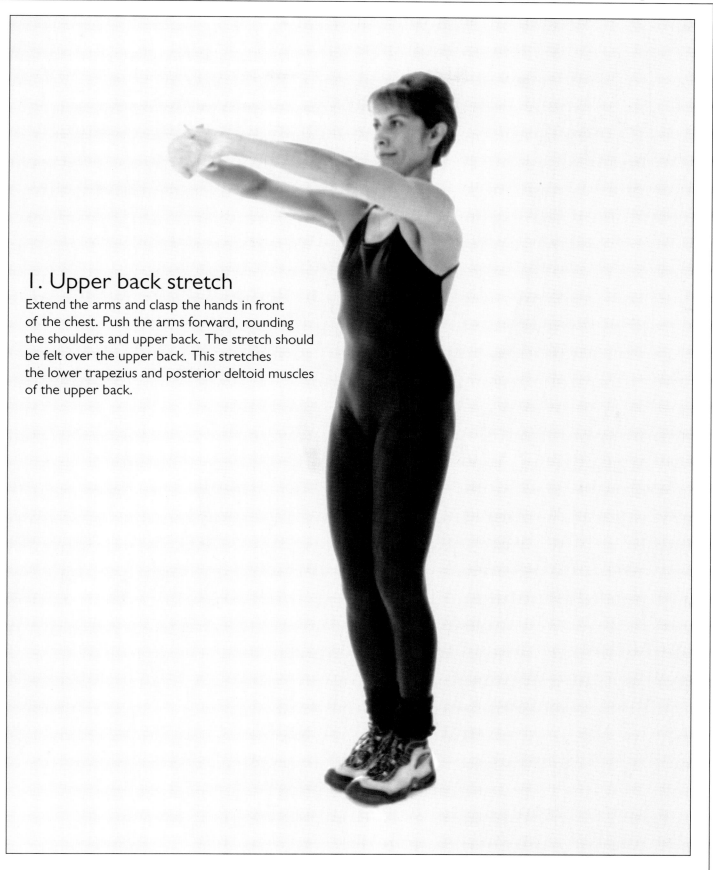

1. Upper back stretch

Extend the arms and clasp the hands in front
of the chest. Push the arms forward, rounding
the shoulders and upper back. The stretch should
be felt over the upper back. This stretches
the lower trapezius and posterior deltoid muscles
of the upper back.

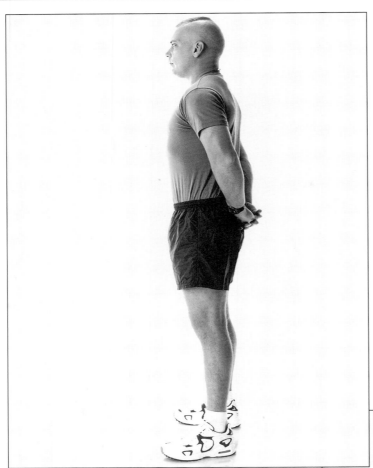

2. Chest stretch

Stand and interlace the fingers behind the back. Pull the arms up toward the head. The stretch should be felt in the front of the chest and shoulders. This stretches the pectoralis major, deltoid, and biceps muscle groups.

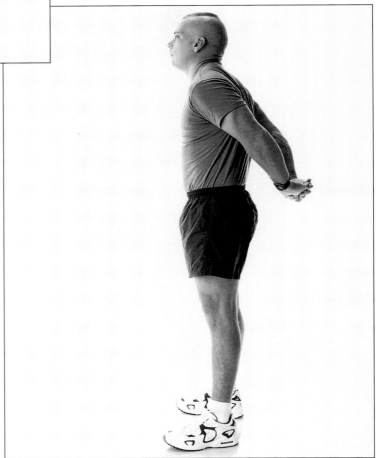

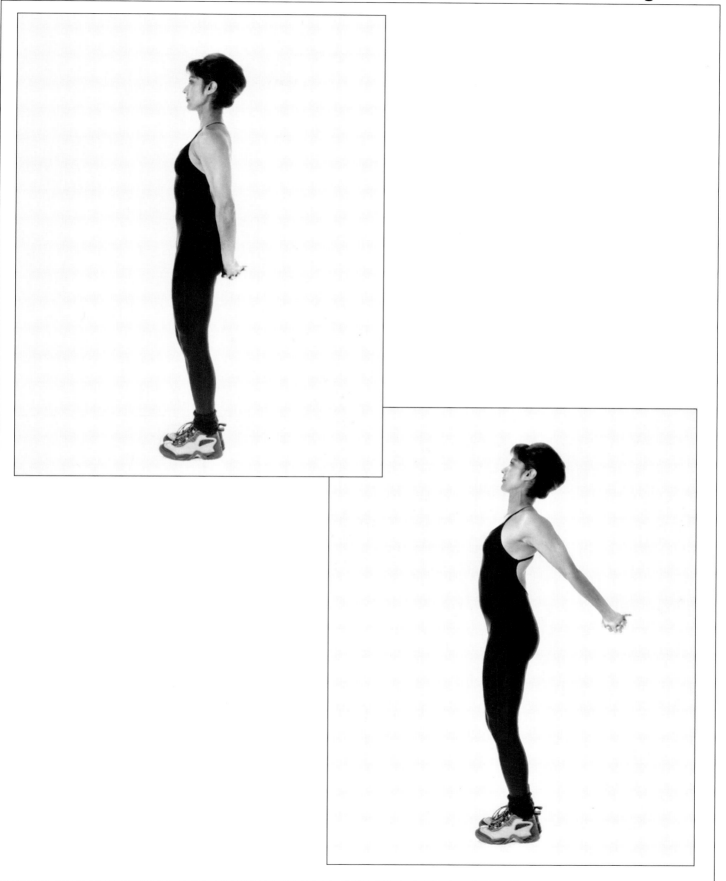

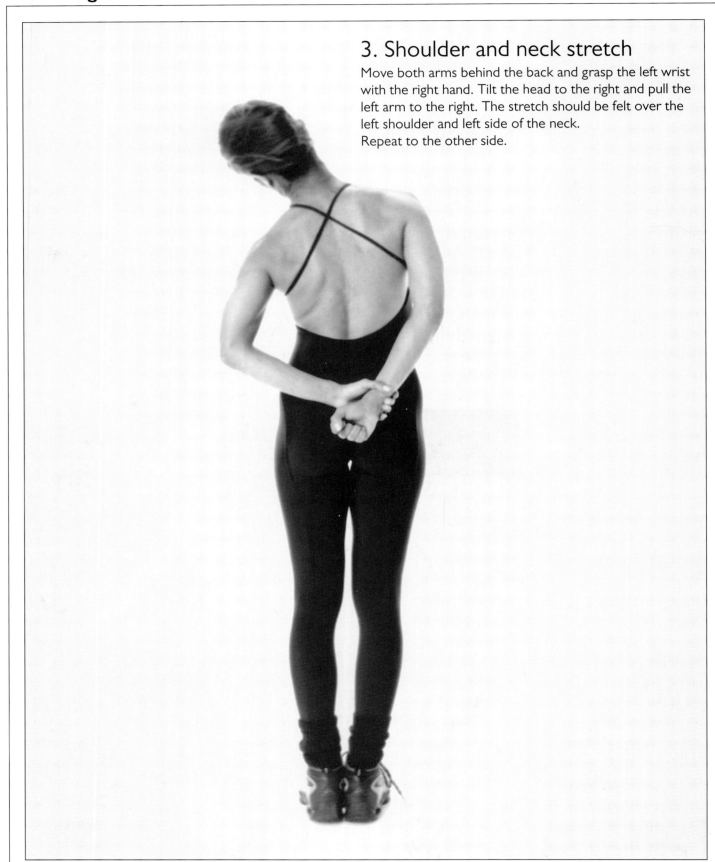

3. Shoulder and neck stretch

Move both arms behind the back and grasp the left wrist with the right hand. Tilt the head to the right and pull the left arm to the right. The stretch should be felt over the left shoulder and left side of the neck.
Repeat to the other side.

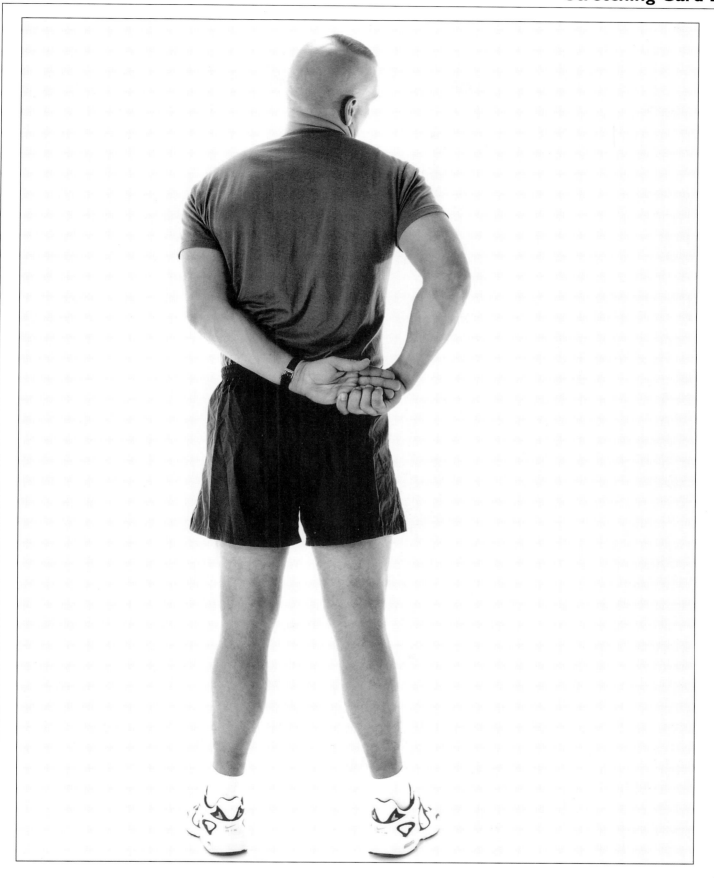

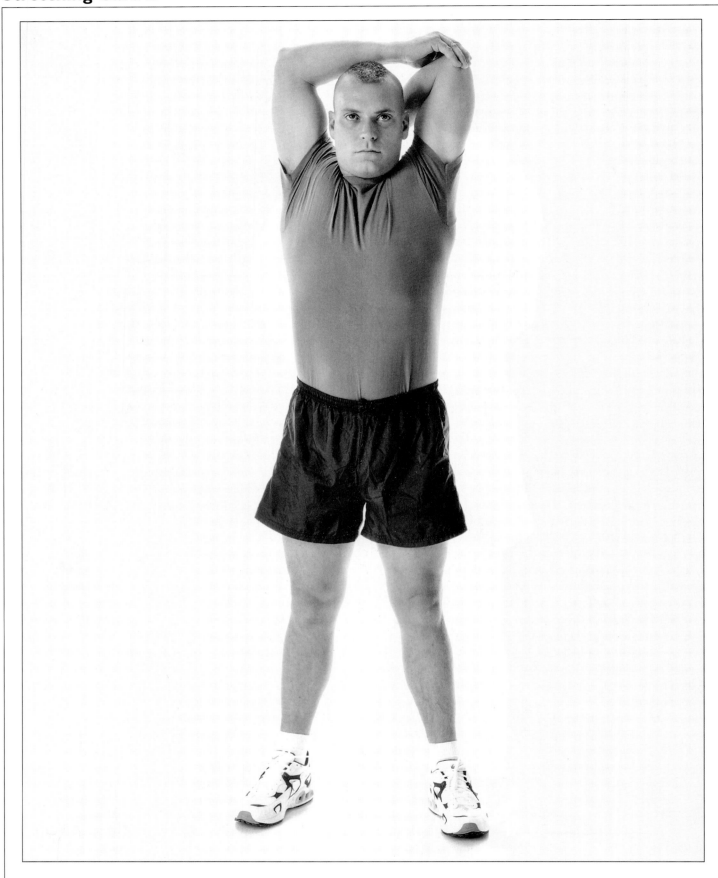

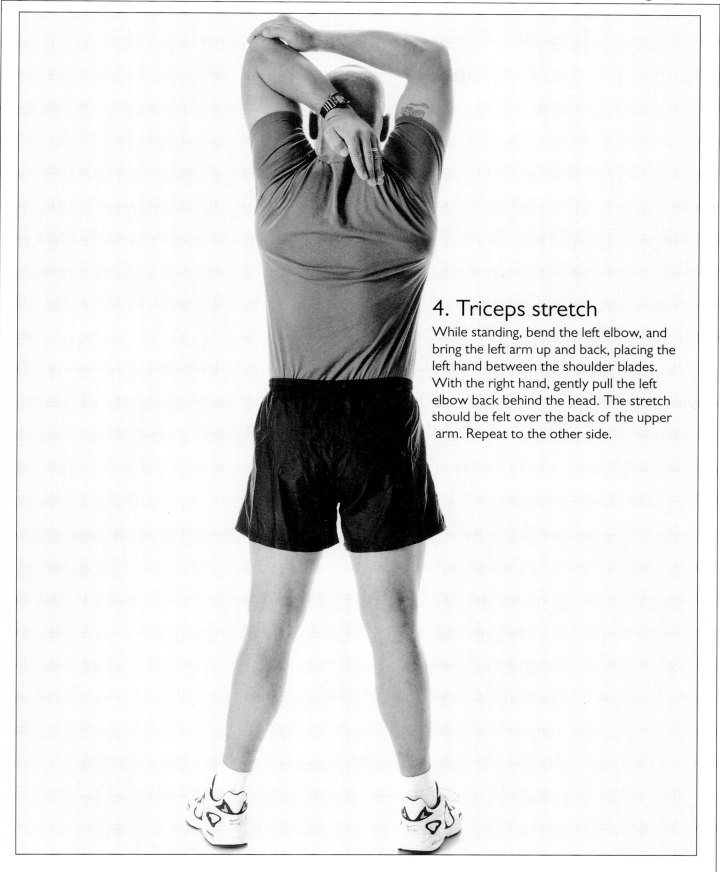

4. Triceps stretch

While standing, bend the left elbow, and bring the left arm up and back, placing the left hand between the shoulder blades. With the right hand, gently pull the left elbow back behind the head. The stretch should be felt over the back of the upper arm. Repeat to the other side.

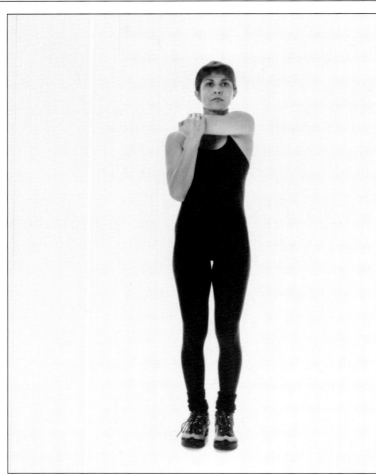

5. Posterior shoulder stretch

Bend the left elbow and bring the left arm across the chest. Give a gentle pull over the posterior left shoulder. Repeat to the other side.

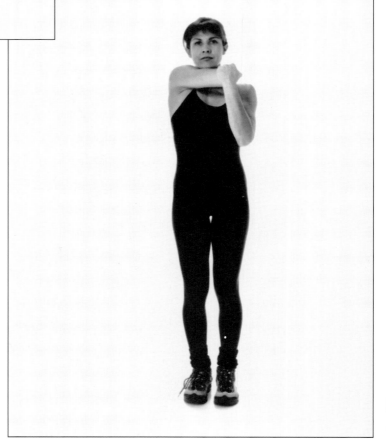

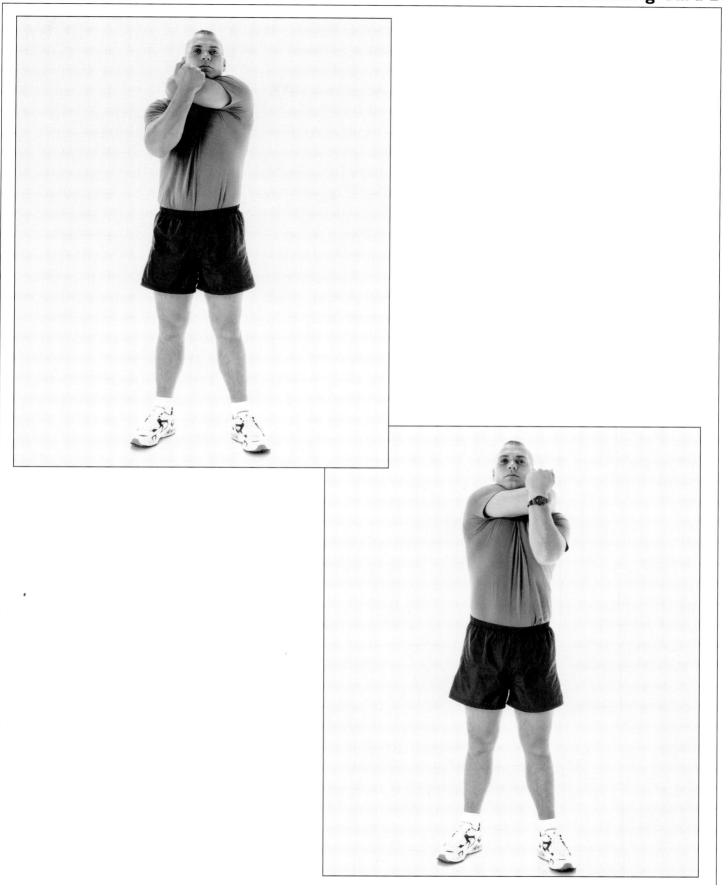

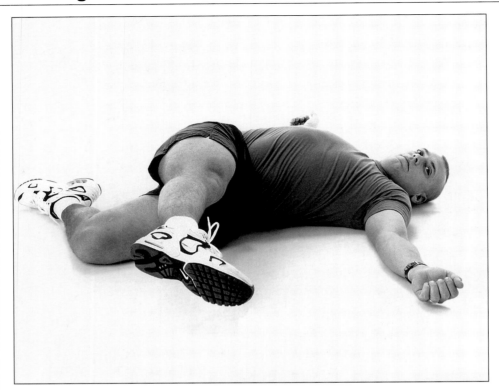

6. Lying down iliotibial band (ITB) stretch

Lying down on the deck, move the left leg until the knee is straight across the body. The stretch should be felt over the left hip. Repeat to the other side.

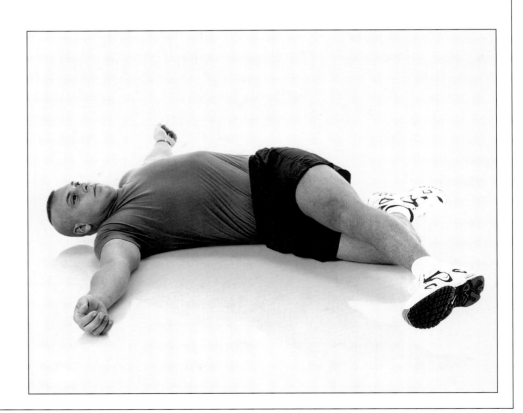

7. Modified hurdler stretch

From a sitting position, extend the left leg out while tucking the right leg in front of the hips with the knee pointing outward. Bend the torso forward toward the left knee. The stretching should be felt over the back of the left thigh. Repeat to the other side.

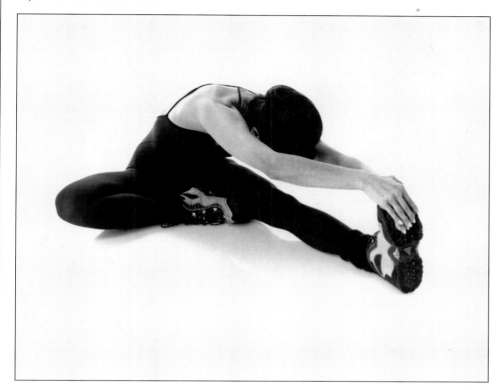

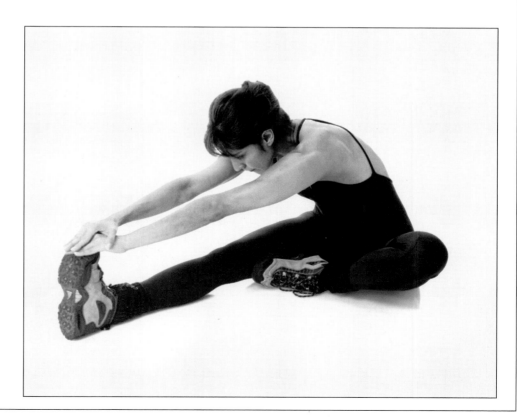

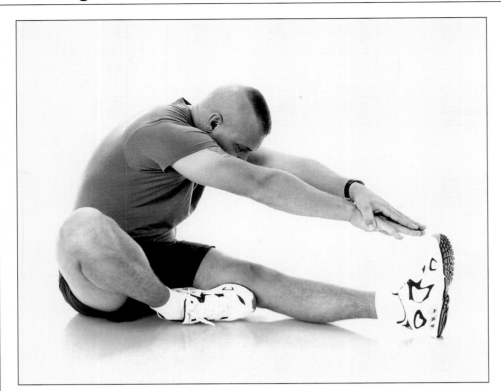

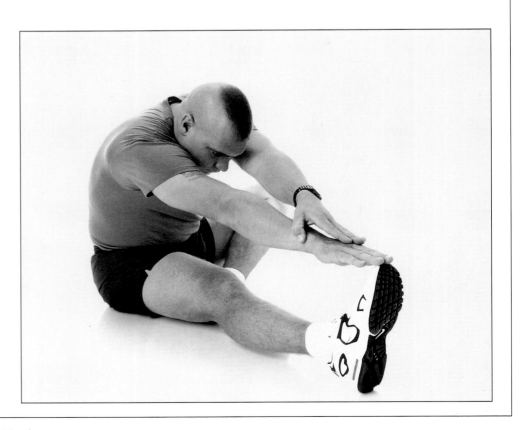

8. Groin stretch

Sit with both knees bent and the bottoms of the feet together. Grasp the feet and gently push knees to the deck with the elbows. The stretch should be felt along the inside of both thighs. Keep the legs as close to the body as possible. This stretches the hip adductor and erector spinae muscles.

NOTE: As you progress, you will be able
to bring your feet closer to your groin.
It is important to keep the back perfectly straight.

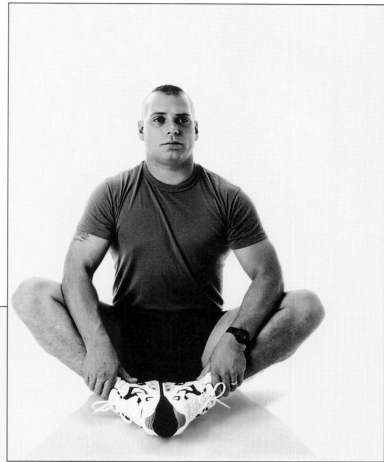

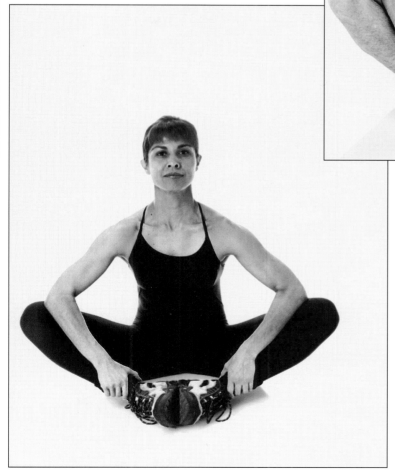

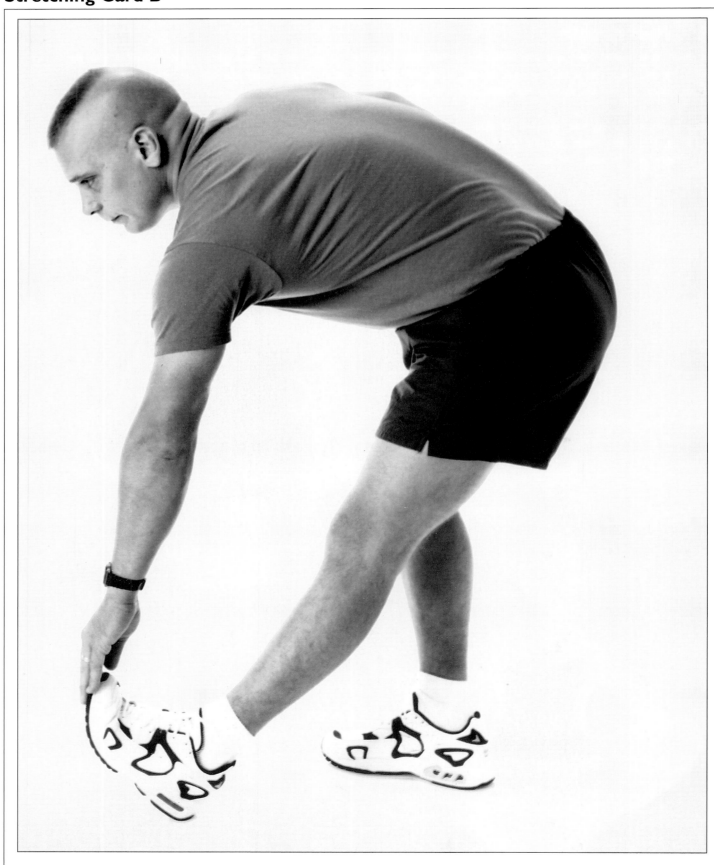

9. Calf stretch

Place the left foot approximately two feet in front of the right foot. Slightly bend the right knee. Lean forward toward the left foot, pointing the left toes up to the sky. If you can grab the left foot, a gentle pull can be given. The stretch should be felt over the left calf. Repeat to the other side. This stretches the calf (gastrocnemius) and, to a lesser extent, the hamstrings, gluteus maximus, and erector spinae muscles.

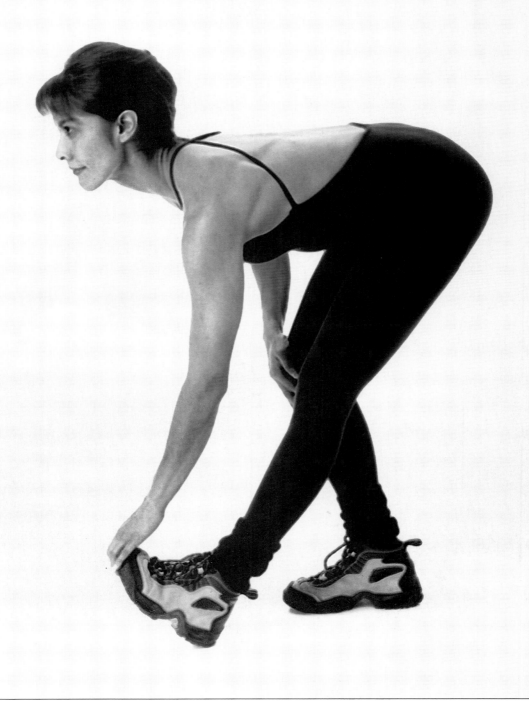

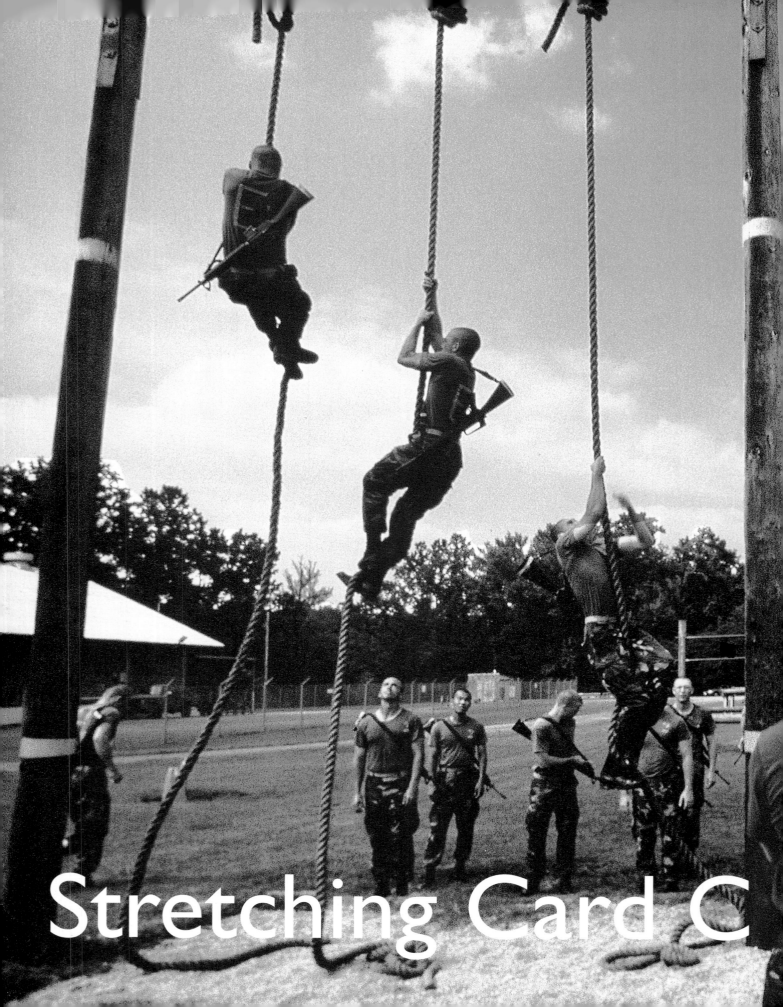

Stretching Card C

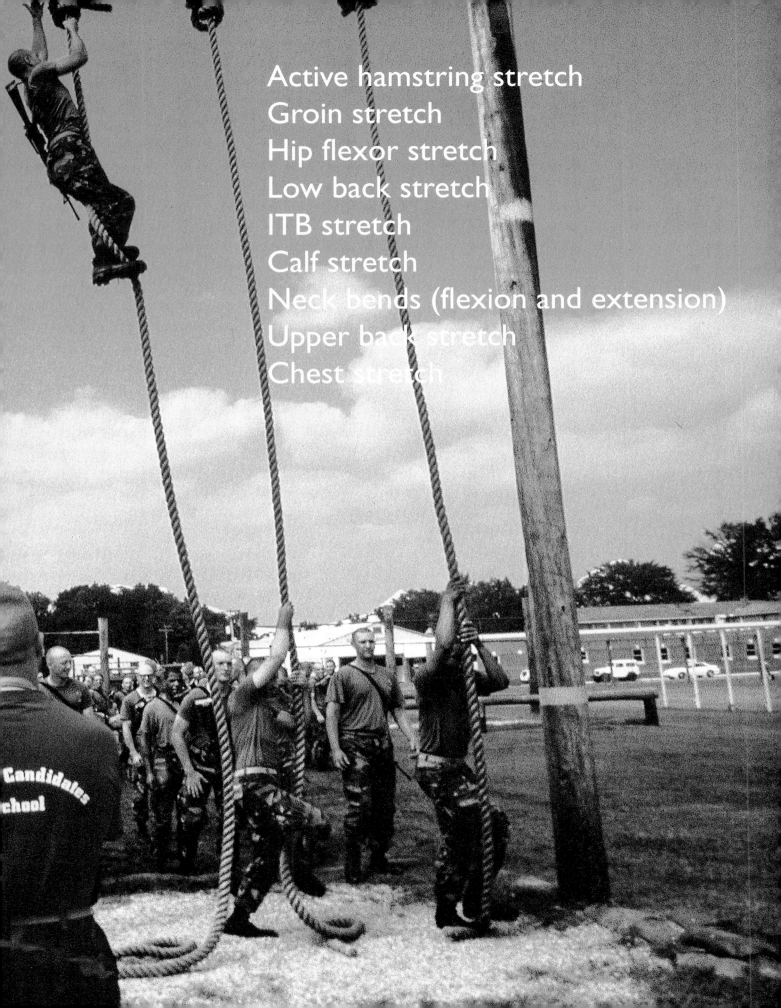

Active hamstring stretch
Groin stretch
Hip flexor stretch
Low back stretch
ITB stretch
Calf stretch
Neck bends (flexion and extension)
Upper back stretch
Chest stretch

Assume all stretching positions slowly until you feel tension or slight discomfort. Hold each position for at least 10 to 15 seconds during the warm-up period. After running, cool-down stretches should be held for approximately 30 seconds.

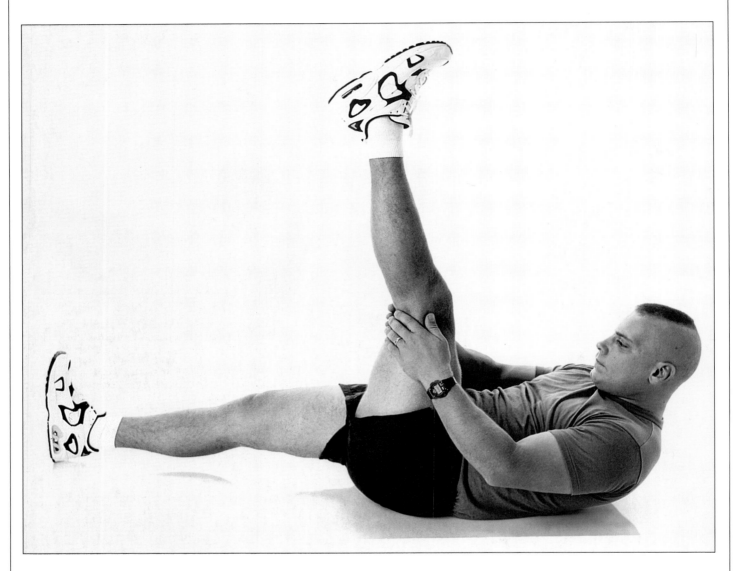

1. Active hamstring stretch

Lying flat on the deck raise left leg 90 degrees. Reach forward with both hands and grasp the leg firmly just below the knee, pulling gently toward the head. Hold for 15 seconds. Repeat on other side. This stretches the hamstrings, erector spinae, gluteal, and calf muscles.

2. Groin stretch

Sit with both knees bent and the bottoms of the feet together. Grasp the feet and gently push knees to the deck with the elbows. The stretch should be felt along the inside of both thighs. Keep the legs as close to the body as possible. This stretches the hip adductor and erector spinae muscles.

NOTE: As you progress you will be able to bring your feet closer to your groin. It is important to keep the back perfectly straight.

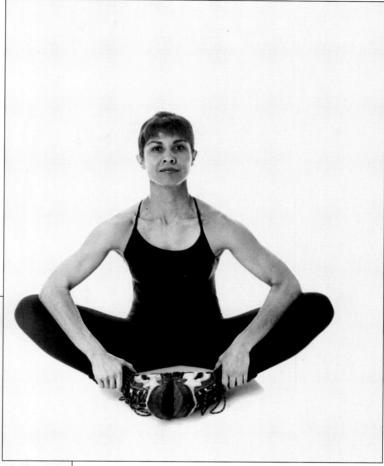

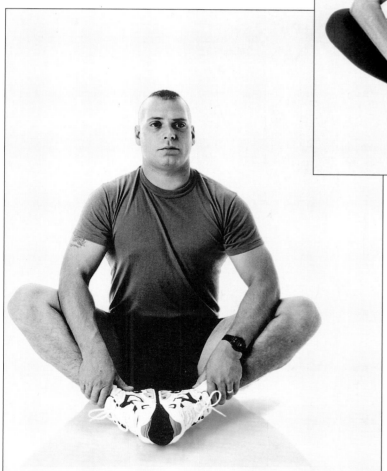

3. Hip flexor stretch

Step the left foot forward three to four feet. Place the right knee on the deck.
Gently move the left knee forward. Place the left hand on
the left knee and the right hand on the right hip.
The stretch should be felt over the
front of the right thigh and hip.
Repeat to the other side.

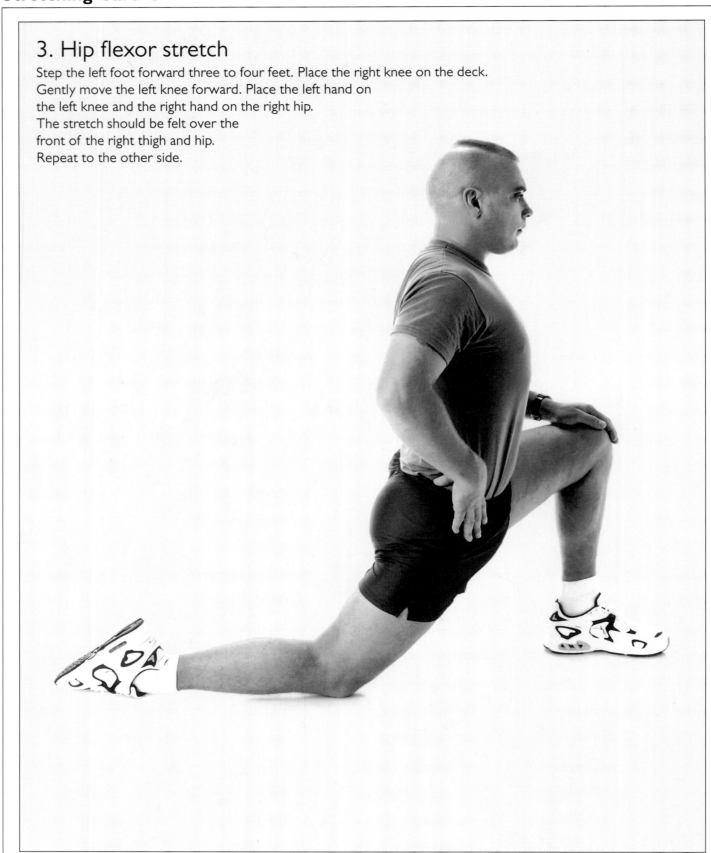

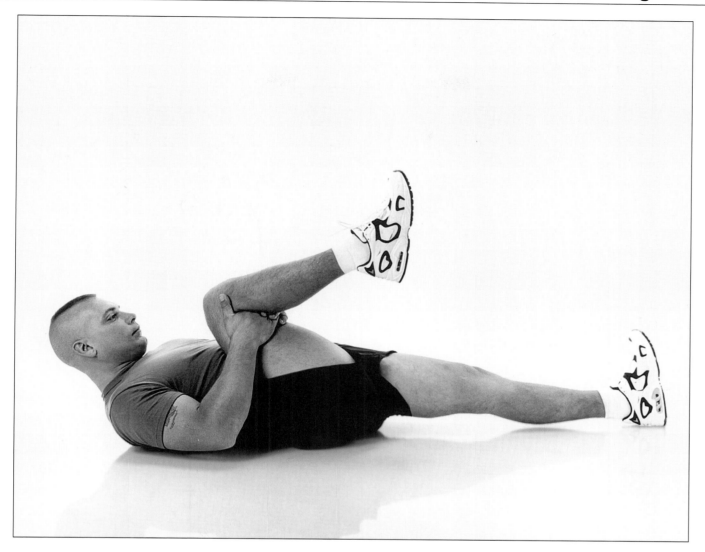

4. Low back stretch

Lying with the back flat against the deck, bring the right knee toward the chest, grasping the right knee. Gently pull the knee tight into the chest. The left leg should remain on the deck. The stretch should be felt along the low back to the right buttock. Repeat to the other side.

NOTE: It is important in this exercise to grab under the thigh and not the knee.

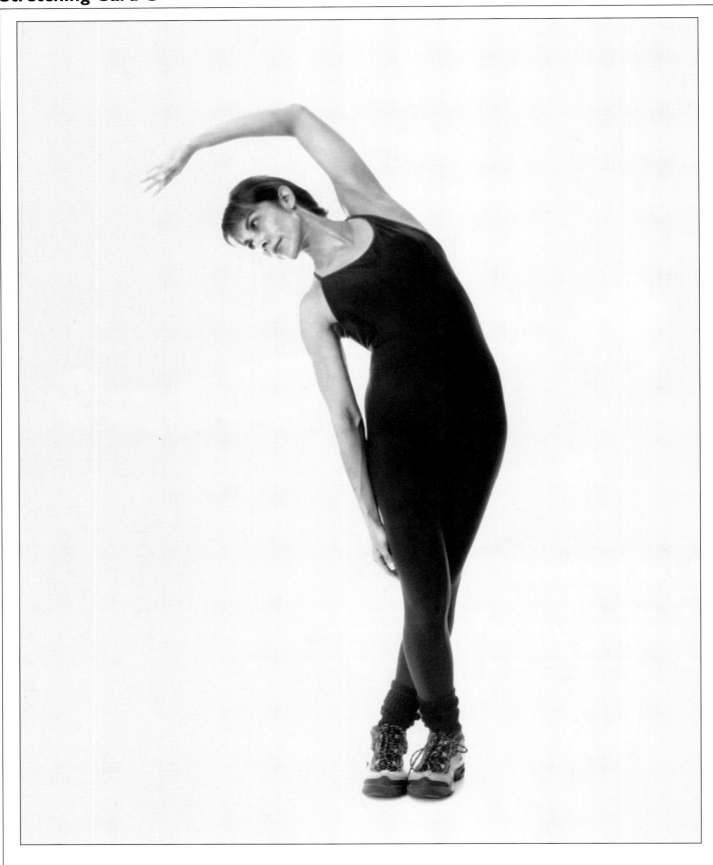

5. Iliotibial band (ITB) stretch

Place the left foot behind and a few inches to the right of the right foot. Bring the left arm over the head. Place body weight on the left leg and bend to the right at the waist. The stretch should be felt over the left hip. Repeat to the other side.

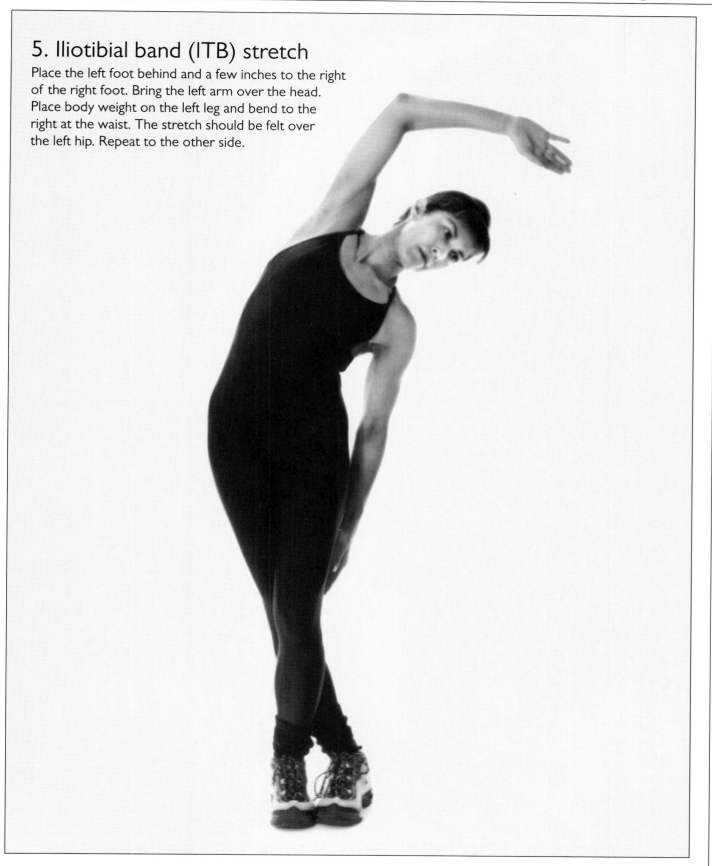

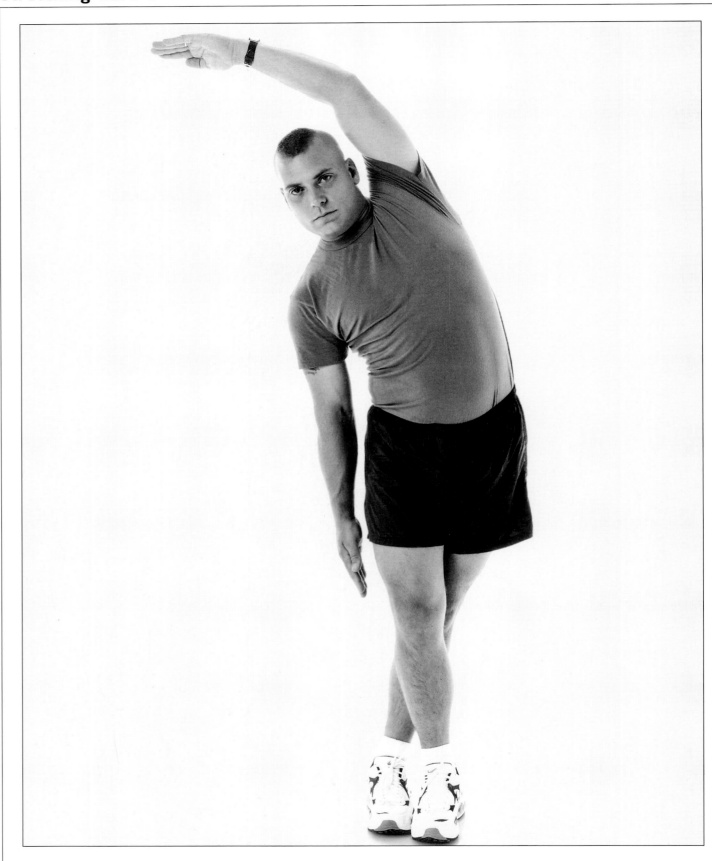

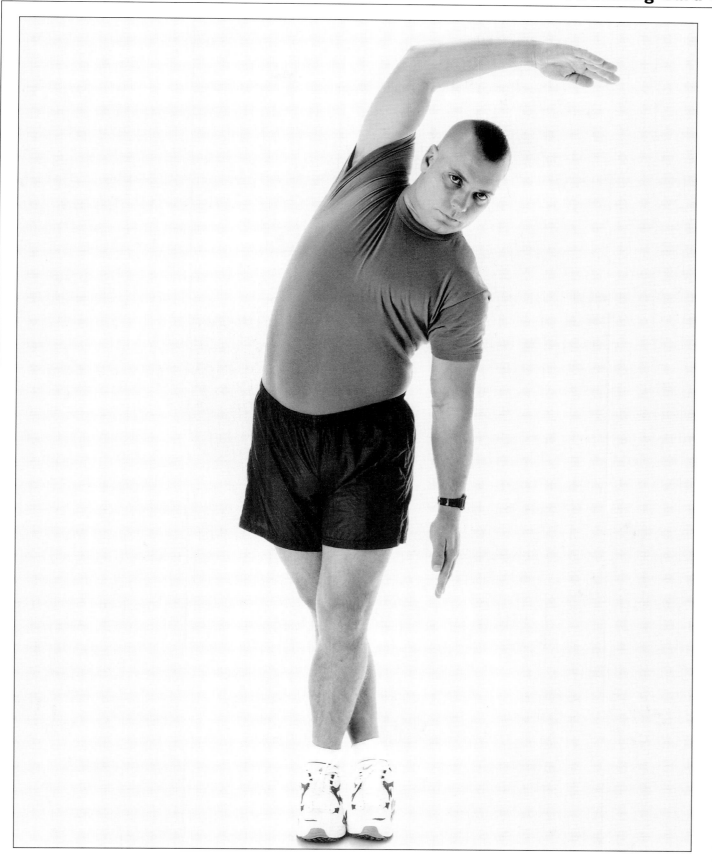

6. Calf stretch (toe-pull)

Place the left foot approximately two feet in front of the right foot. Slightly bend the right knee. Lean forward toward the left foot, pointing the left toes up to the sky. If you can grab the left foot, a gentle pull can be given. The stretch should be felt over the left calf. Repeat to the other side. This stretches the calf (gastrocnemius) and, to a lesser extent, the hamstrings, gluteus maximus, and erector spinae muscles.

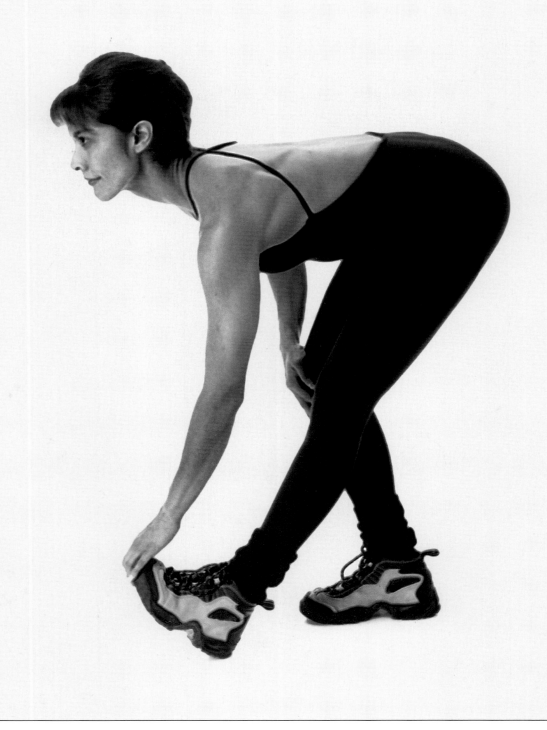

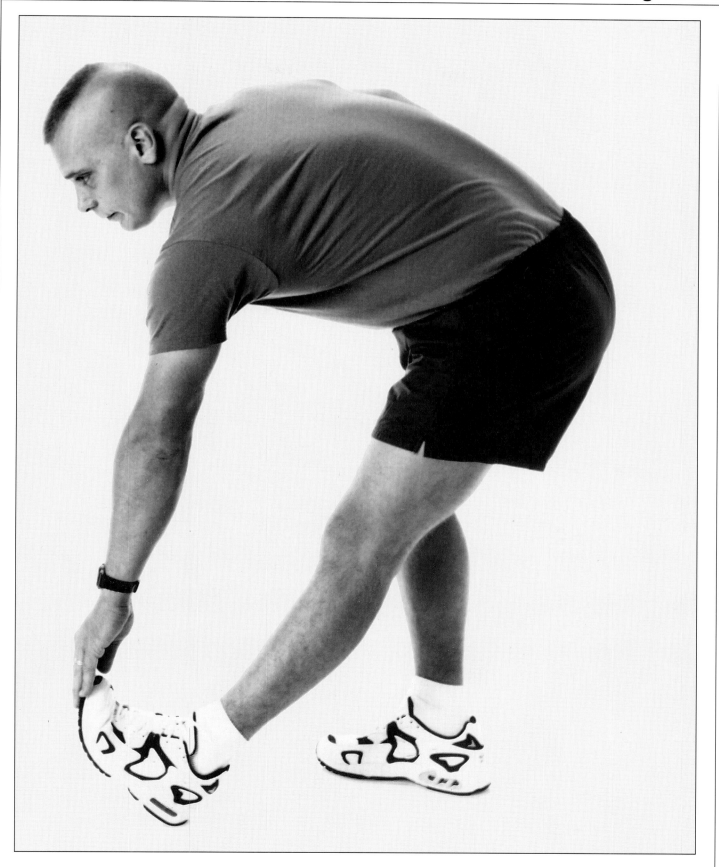

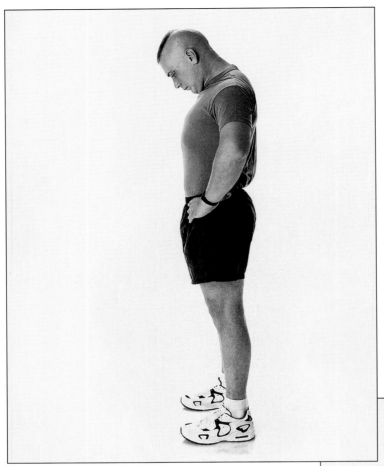

7. Neck bends

Neck bend (front to back)

Flex the neck forward, bringing the chin toward the chest. Extend the head back.
Five to 10 repetitions.

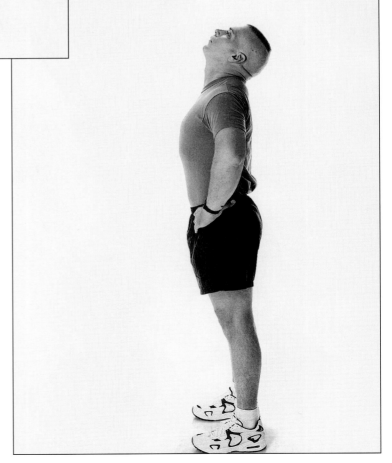

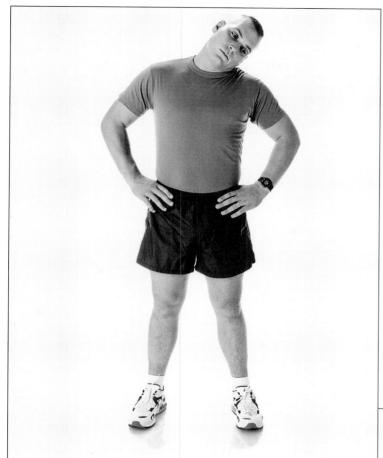

Neck bend (side to side)

Tilt the head to the left side, bringing the left ear toward the left shoulder. Repeat to the right side. Five to 10 repetitions.

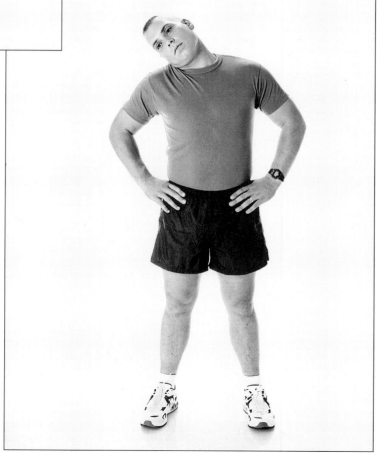

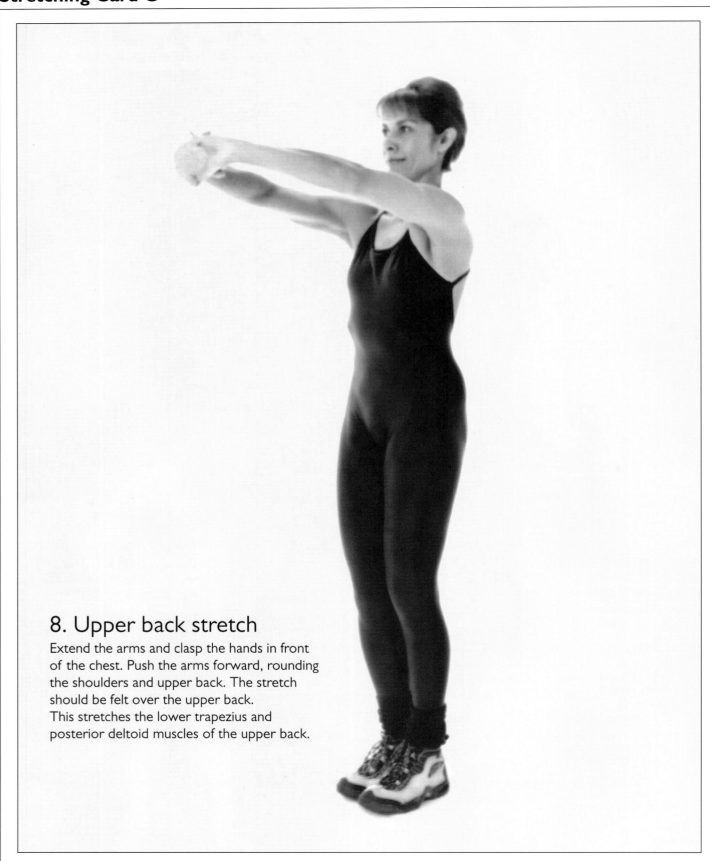

8. Upper back stretch

Extend the arms and clasp the hands in front
of the chest. Push the arms forward, rounding
the shoulders and upper back. The stretch
should be felt over the upper back.
This stretches the lower trapezius and
posterior deltoid muscles of the upper back.

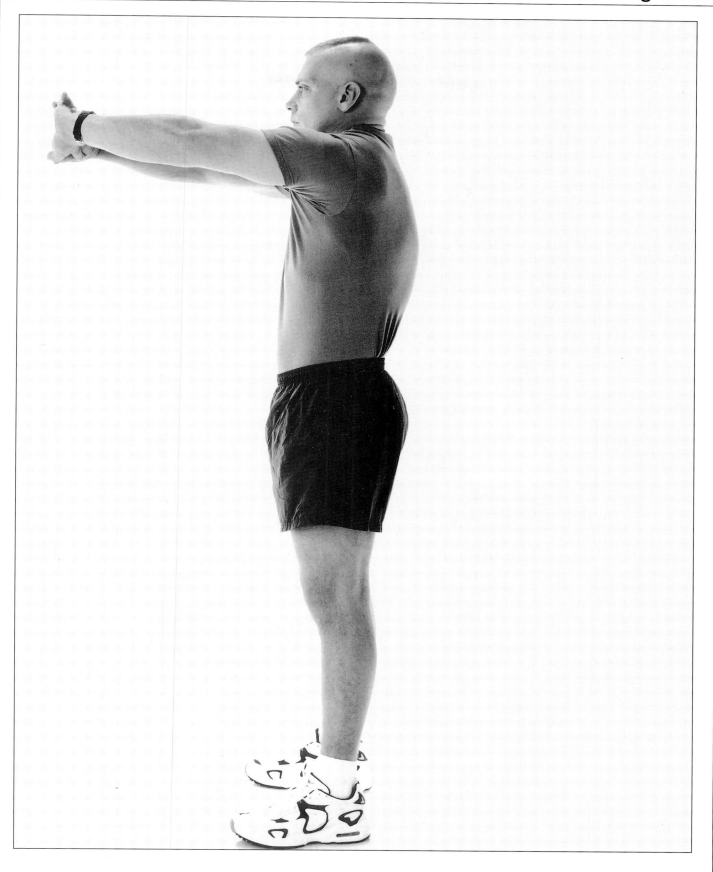

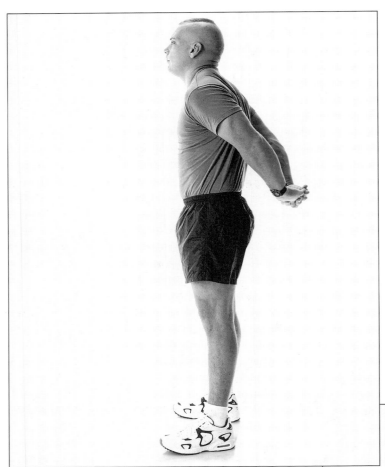

9. Chest stretch

Stand and interlace the fingers behind the back. Pull the arms up toward the head. The stretch should be felt in the front of the chest and shoulders. This stretches the pectoralis major, deltoid, and biceps muscle groups.

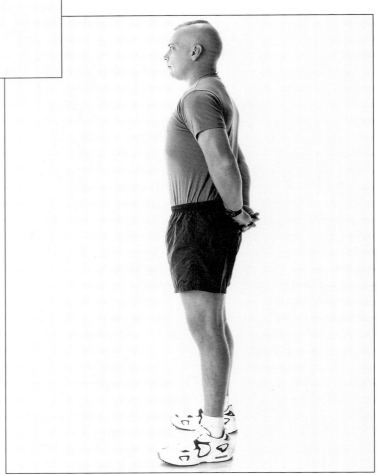

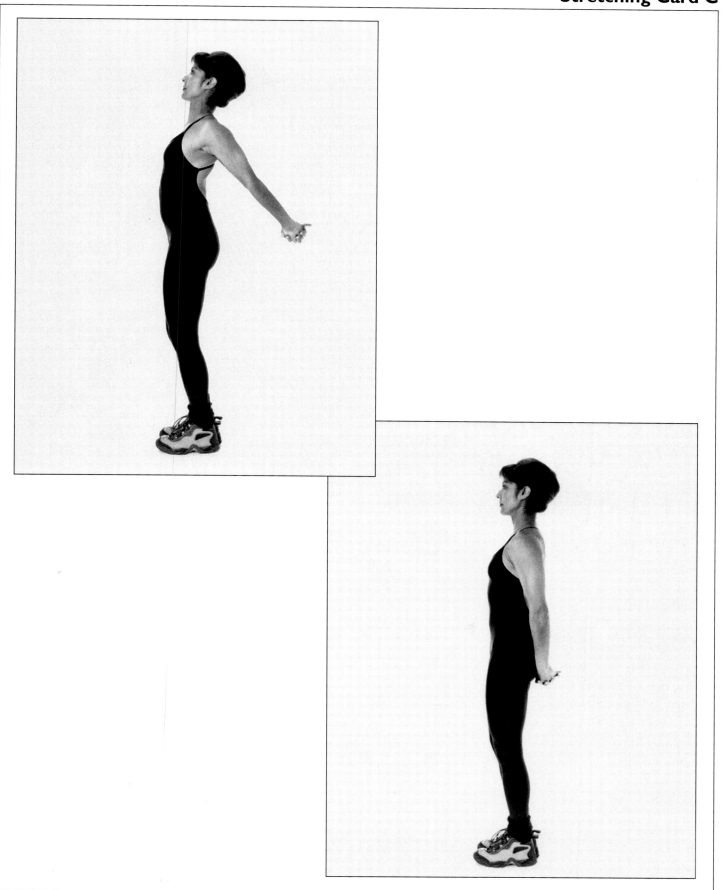

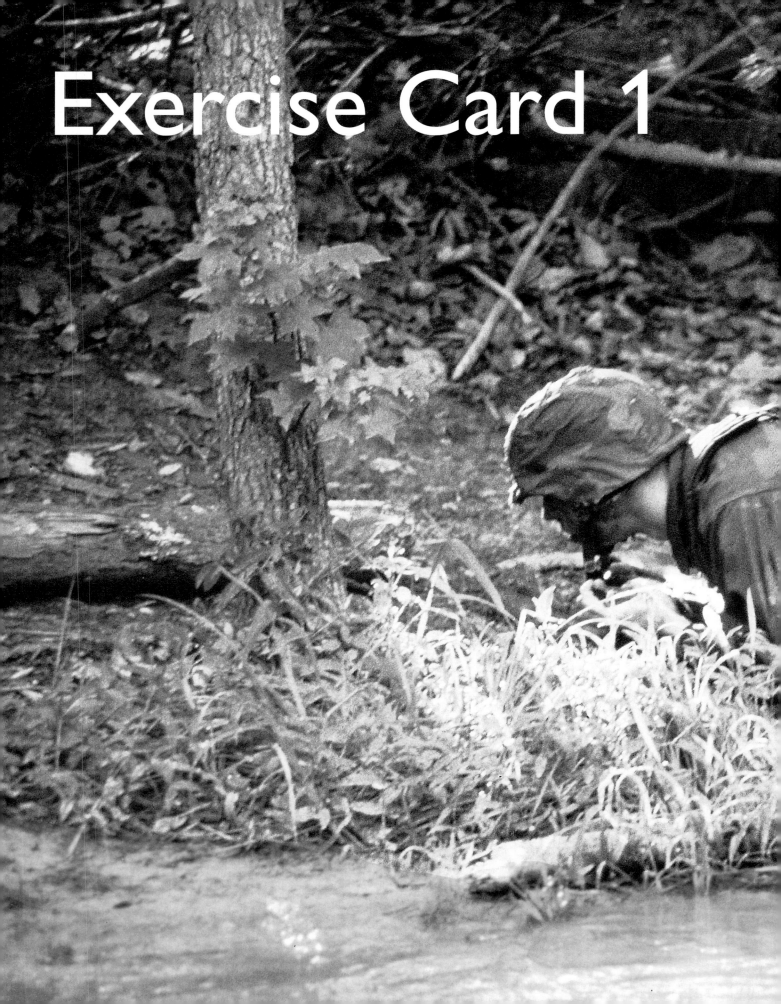

Exercise Card 1

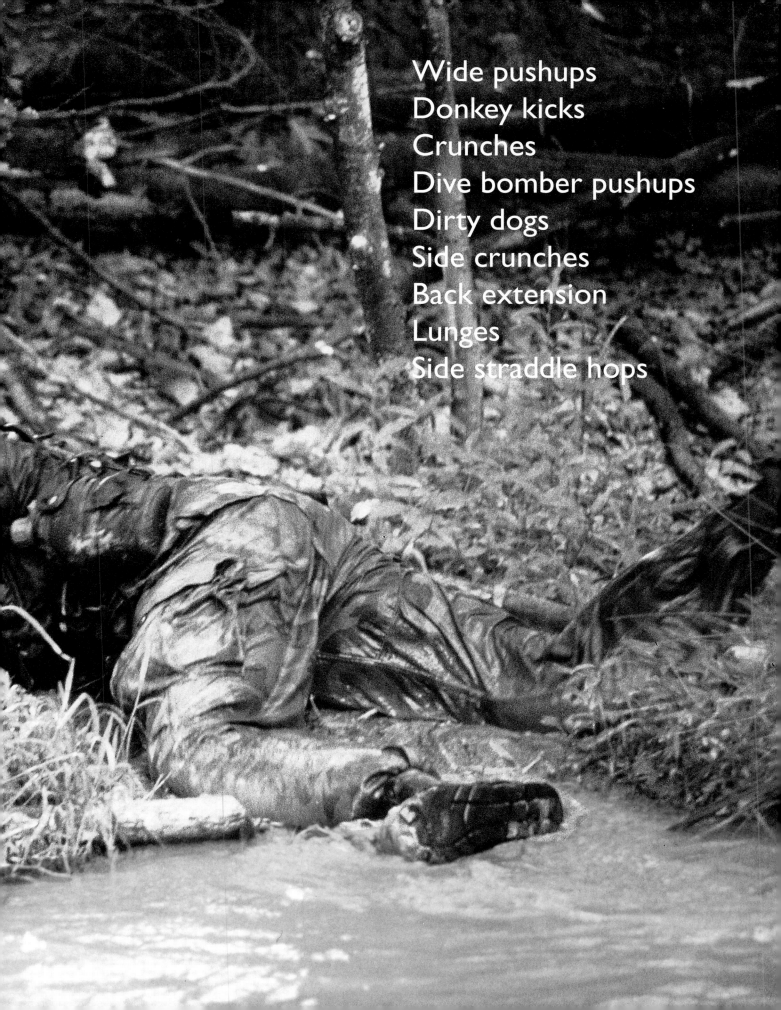

Wide pushups
Donkey kicks
Crunches
Dive bomber pushups
Dirty dogs
Side crunches
Back extension
Lunges
Side straddle hops

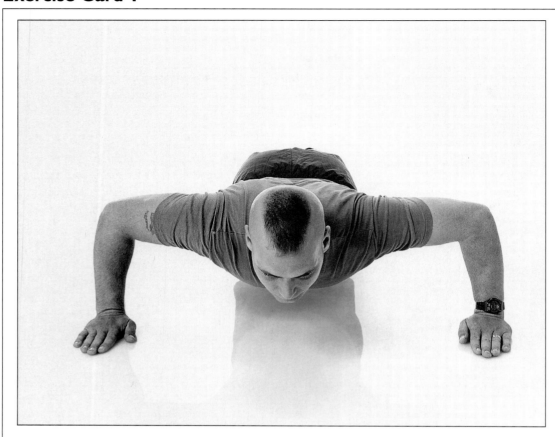

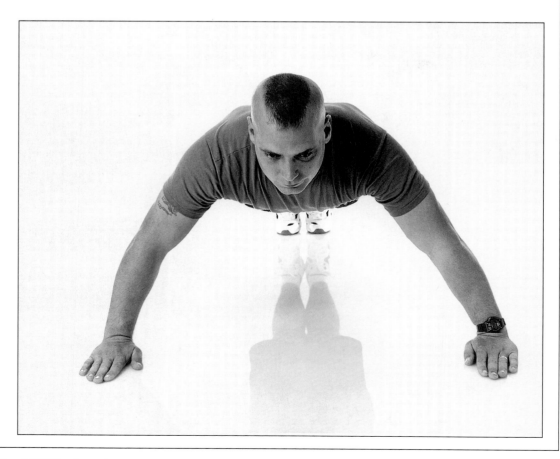

1. Wide pushups

Start in down pushup position with hands spread beyond shoulder width. Push up until the elbows are fully extended. On the first and third count, lower the chest to the deck, bending the elbows to at least 90 degrees. On the second and fourth count, extend the arms back to the starting position. This exercise conditions the chest and anterior shoulder primarily and secondarily the triceps. With the wider hand position, the chest muscles increase their workload. Five to 10 repetitions.

NOTE: It is key that the chest and stomach never touch the deck.

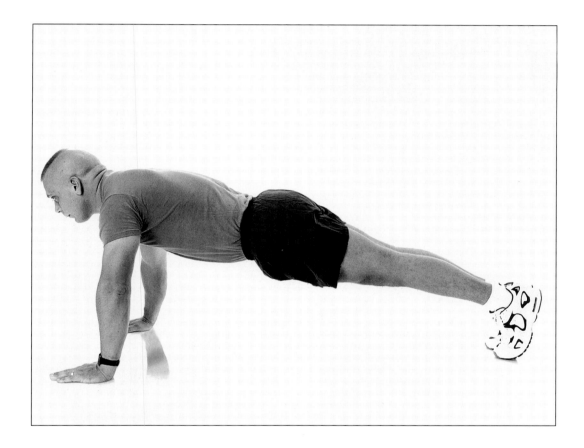

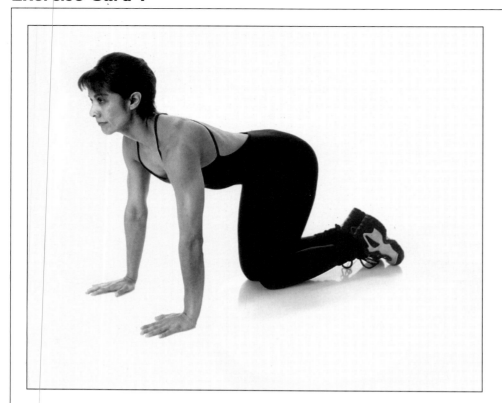

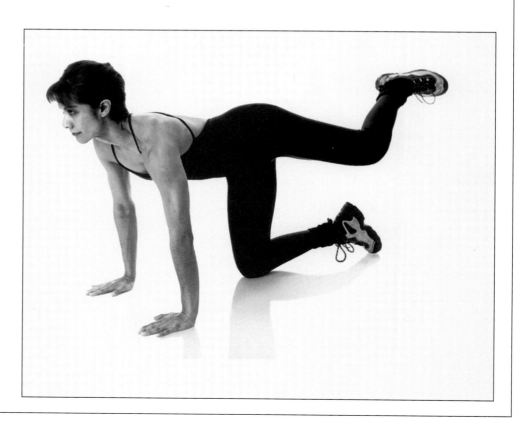

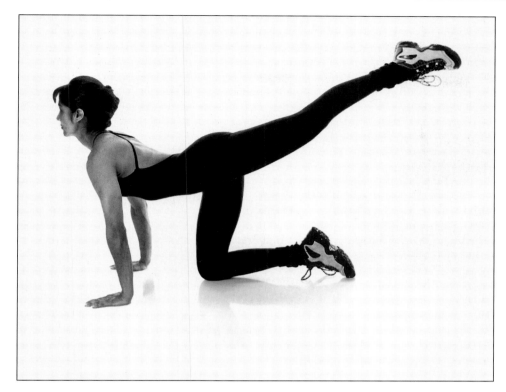

2. Donkey kicks

Start on the hands and knees. On the first and third count, kick the left leg back and up, straightening the knee. On the second and fourth count, bend the knee and hip, bringing the left knee into the chest. The back should not hyperextend during this exercise. Repeat to the other side. Five to 10 repetitions. This exercise conditions the muscles that extend the hip.

NOTE: Make kick and recovery separate motions, rather than getting into a continuous swing.

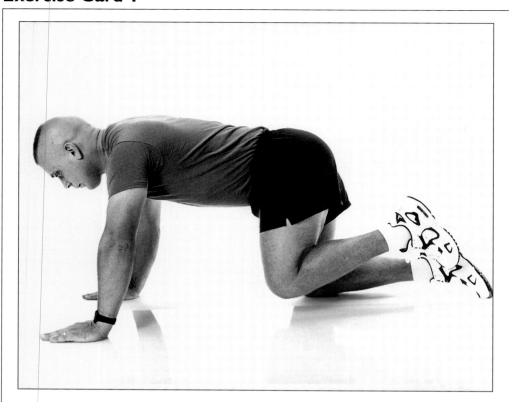

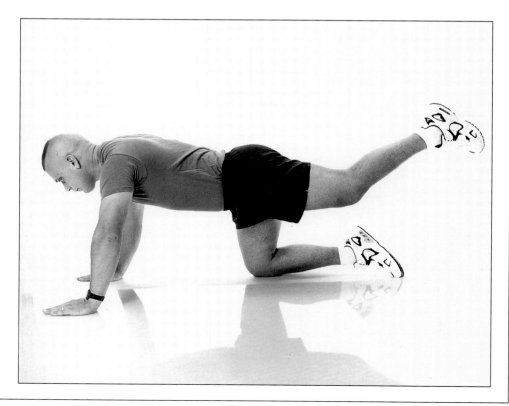

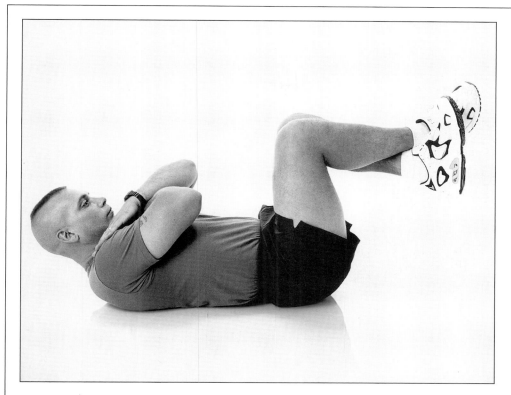

3. Crunches

Start on the back with hips bent to 90 degrees and knees bent, feet off the ground. Bend the elbows to 90 degrees and fold across the chest. On the first and third count, raise the upper torso off the deck, touching the thighs with the forearms. When coming forward, it is not essential to touch the knees with the forearms. Come as close as you can. Make sure the chin remains on the chest. On the second and fourth count, return to the starting position. This should be done in a slow and controlled manner. This exercise conditions the abdominal muscles. Five to 10 repetitions.

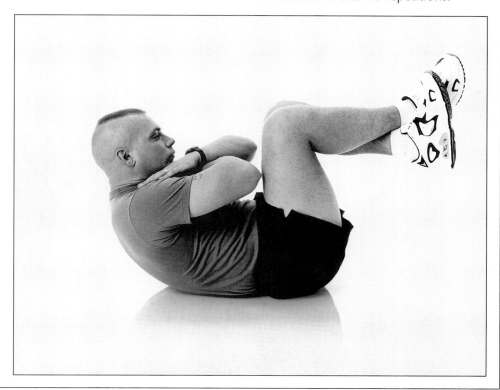

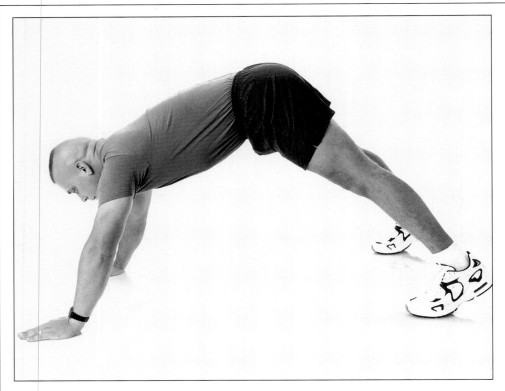

4. Dive bomber pushups

Start in basic up pushup position with hands and toes on the ground with elbows and knees straight. The hands and feet will extend beyond shoulder width, except that the hips will be raised up, the butt raised, and the shoulders behind the hands.

On the second count, continue to move torso forward, extending the elbows so that now the shoulders are in front of the hands.

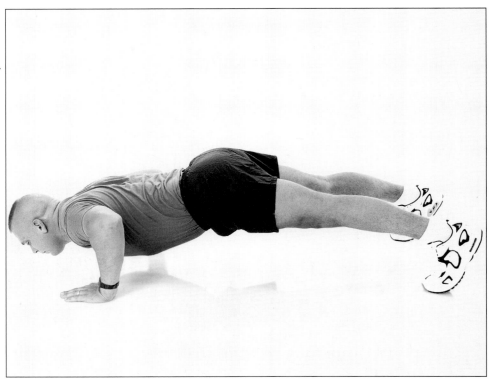

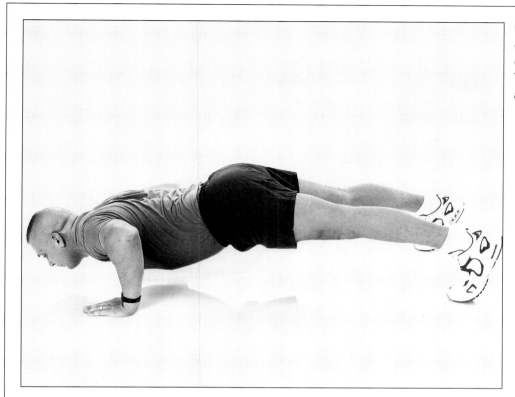

On the third count, reverse torso direction to the rear, lowering the chest down and back to the deck. The shoulders will be directly over the hands.

On the fourth count, continue to rock back up to the starting position. This is done in a smooth, rhythmic motion. This exercise primarily conditions the chest and anterior shoulder and, secondarily, the triceps. Five to 10 repetitions.

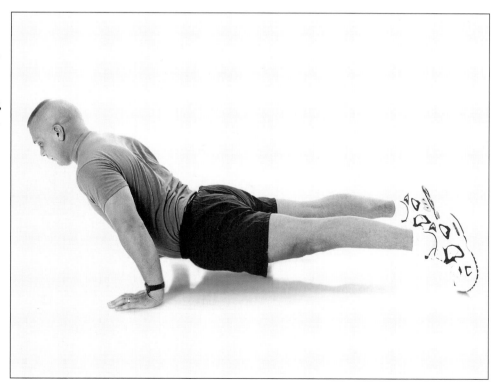

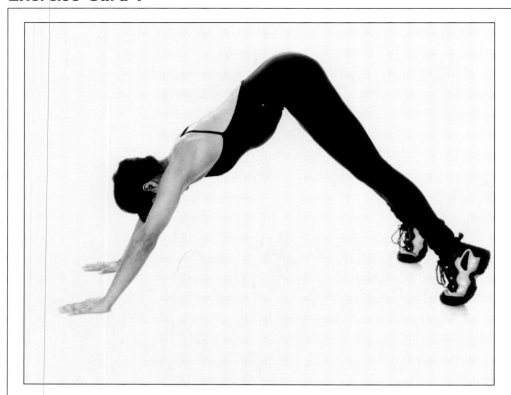

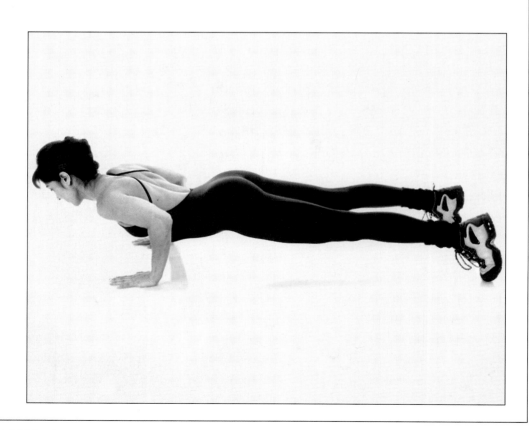

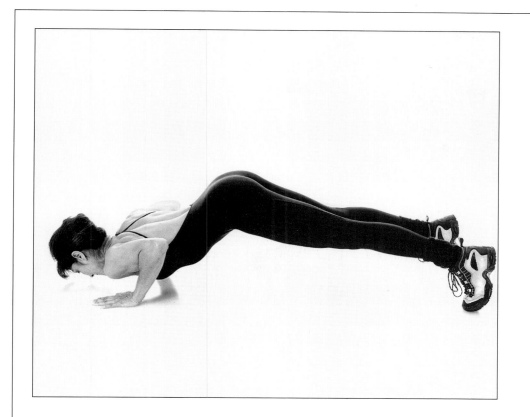

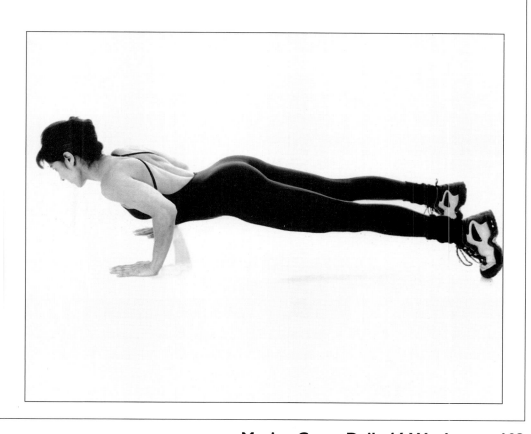

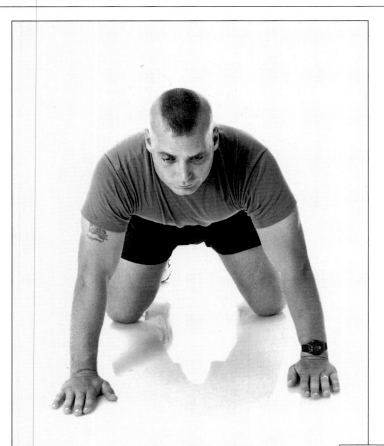

5. Dirty dogs

Start on the hands and knees.

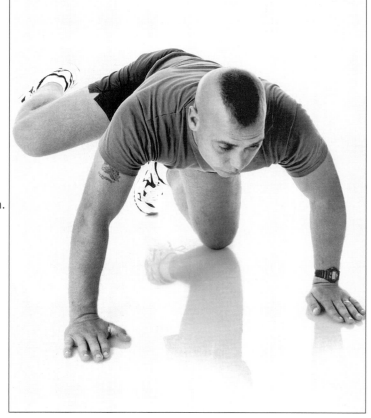

On the first and third count, raise the right leg to the side, while keeping the knee bent. On the second and fourth count, return the leg to the starting position. Repeat to the other side. This exercise conditions the hip abductors. Five to 10 repetitions.

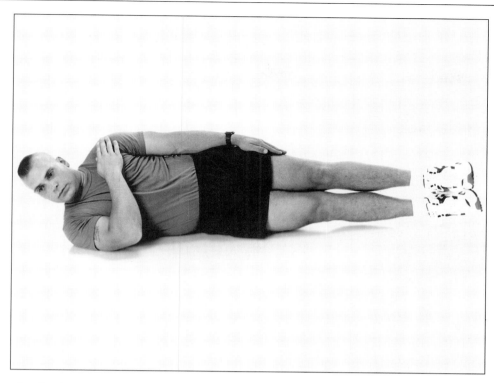

6. Side crunches

Start on the right side with the right arm across the chest and left arm along the side of the body. On the first and third count, raise the upper torso and feet off the deck, sliding the right hand down the thigh. On the second and fourth count, return to the starting position. Repeat to the other side. This exercise conditions the abdominal muscles with emphasis on the obliques. Five to 10 repetitions.

NOTE: Be careful not to bring the shoulder all the way down to the deck.

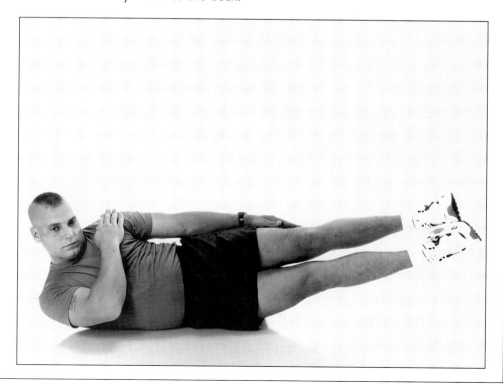

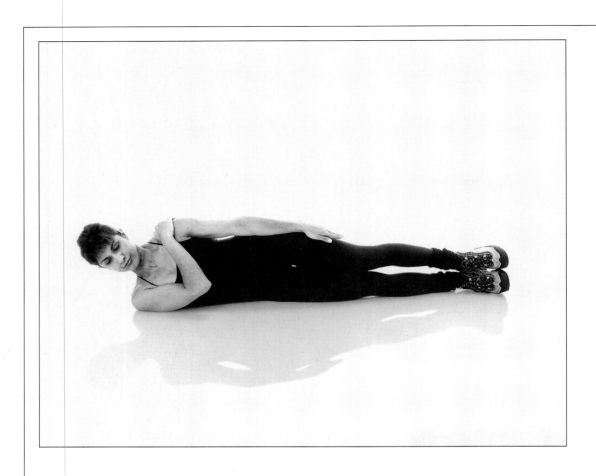

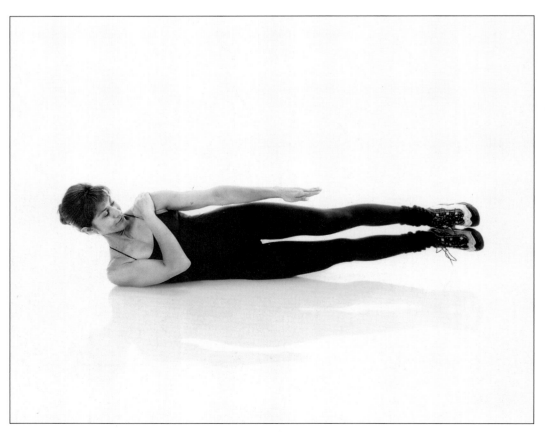

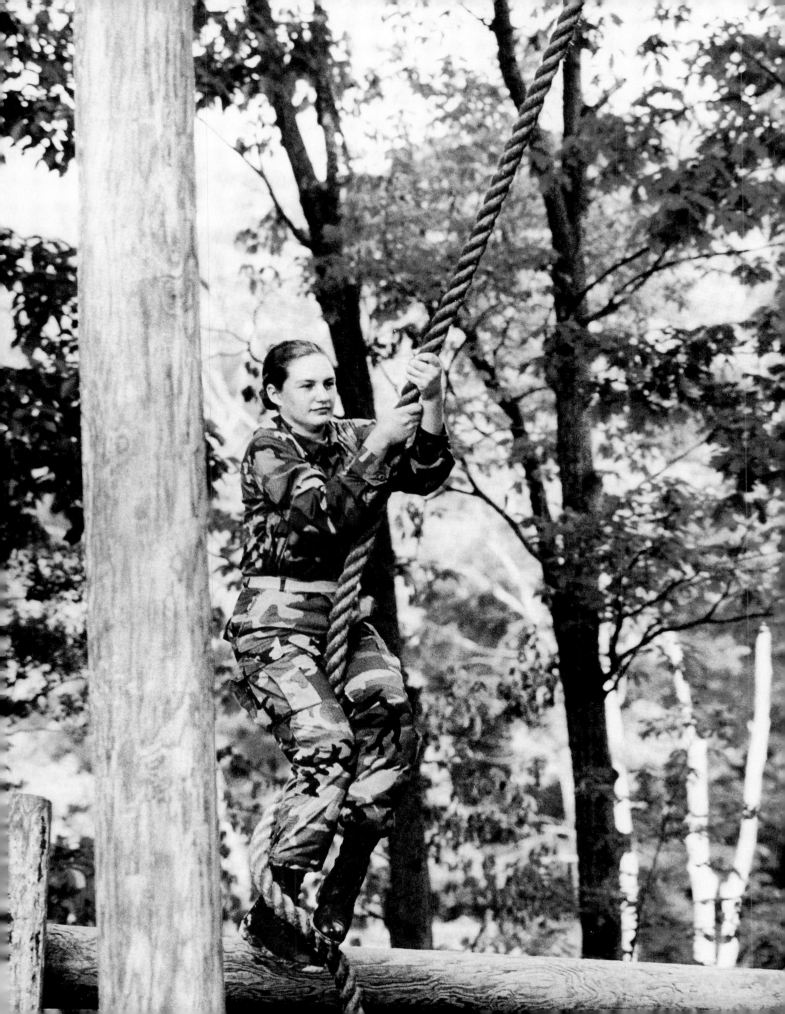

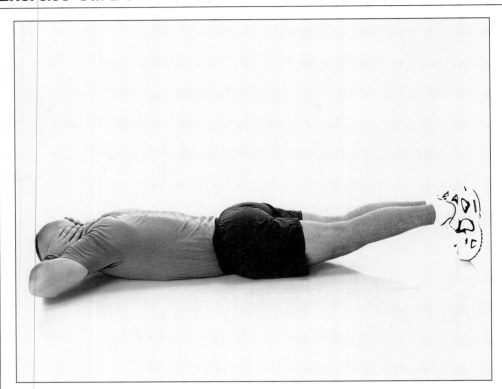

7. Back extension

Start on the stomach with the hands behind the head. On the first and third count, raise the upper torso and legs off the deck. On the second and fourth count, lower the upper torso and legs to the starting position. This exercise conditions the muscles that extend the back. Five to 10 repetitions.

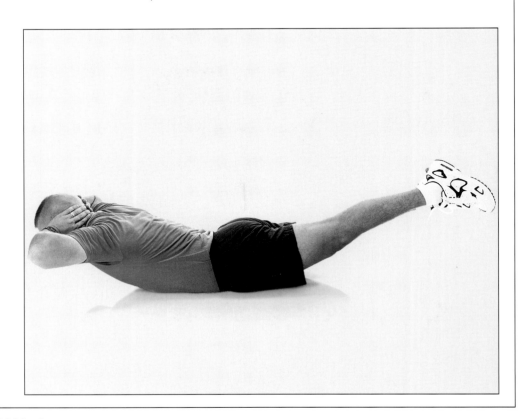

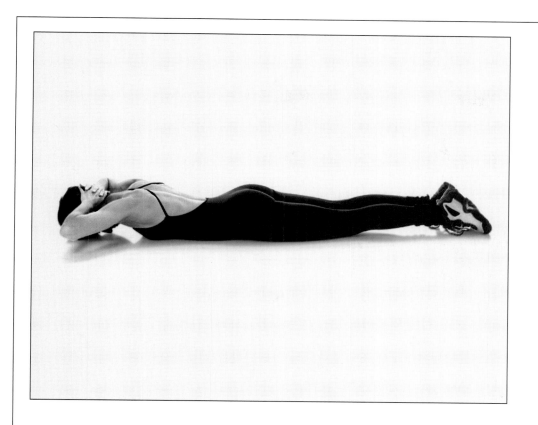

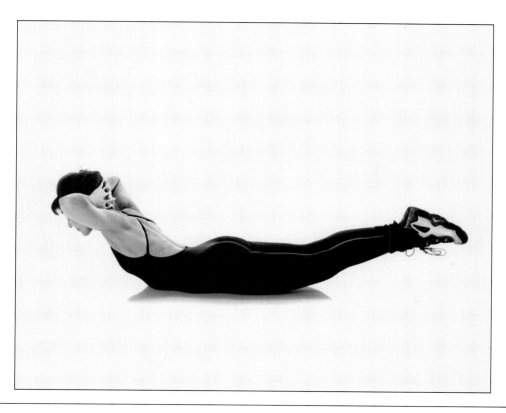

8. Lunges

Start standing with the feet shoulder-width apart and hands on the hips. On the first count, touch the right knee to the deck by stepping forward with the left foot and bending knees. On the second count, return to the starting position. On the third count, touch the left knee to the deck by stepping forward with the right foot and bending both knees. On the fourth count, return to the starting position. Do not bend the forward knee beyond the toes. Do in a controlled cadence. This exercise conditions the muscles that extend the hip and knee of the forward leg.
Five to 10 repetitions.

NOTE: It is important to keep the back as straight as possible.

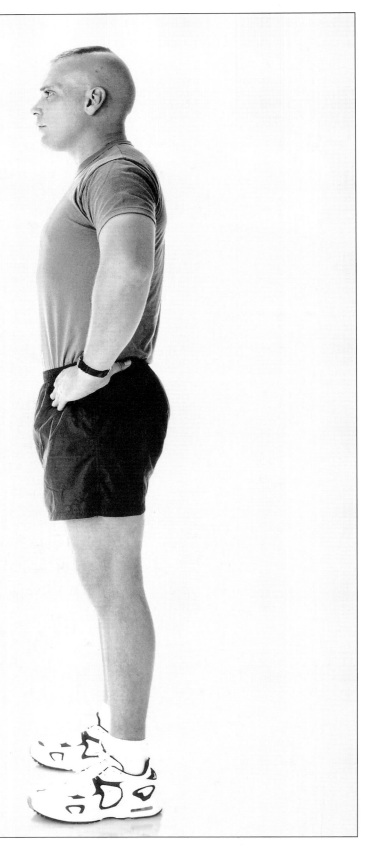

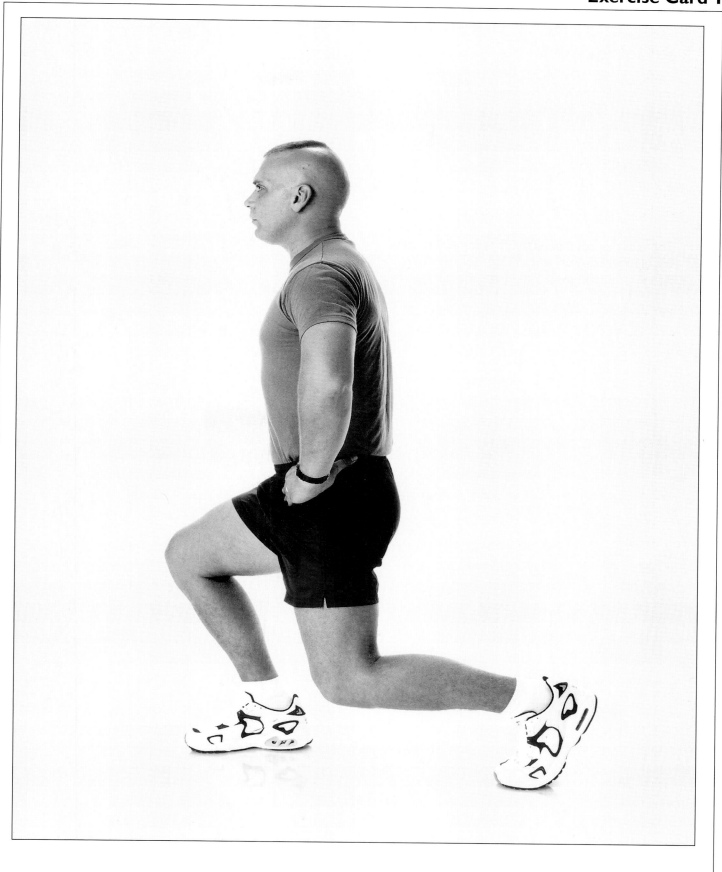

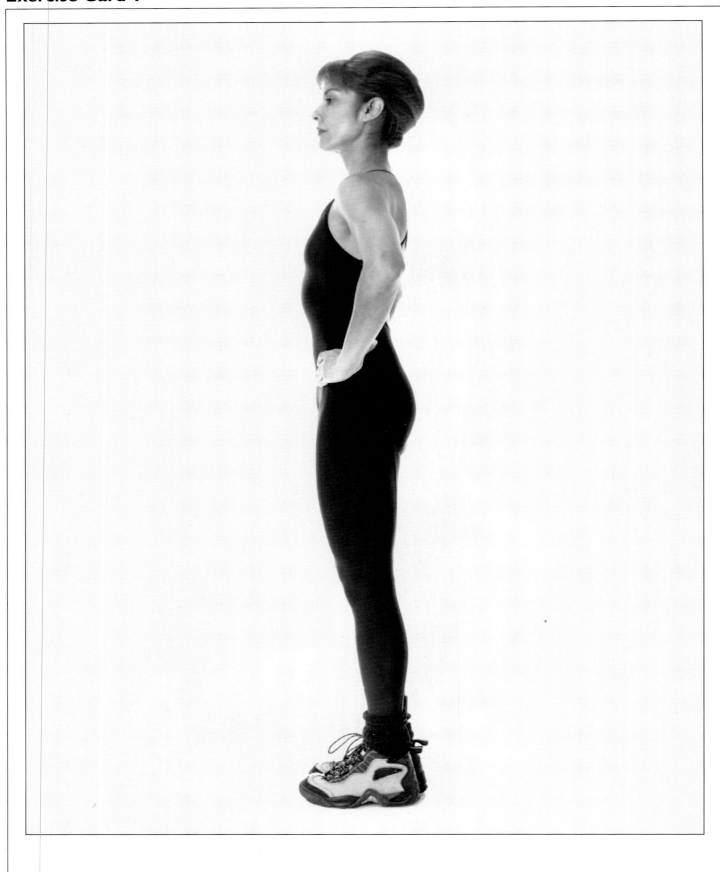

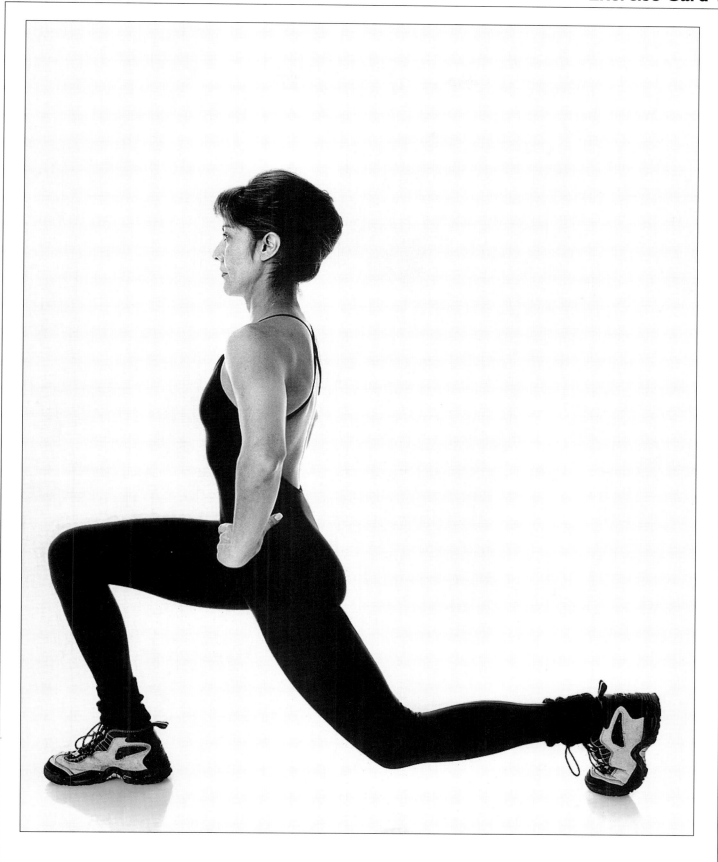

9. Side-straddle hops

Stand erect with the feet together and arms at the sides. On the first and third count, jump and land with the feet just beyond shoulder width apart while bringing the hands together overhead. On the second and fourth count, jump back to the starting position. Five to 10 repetitions.

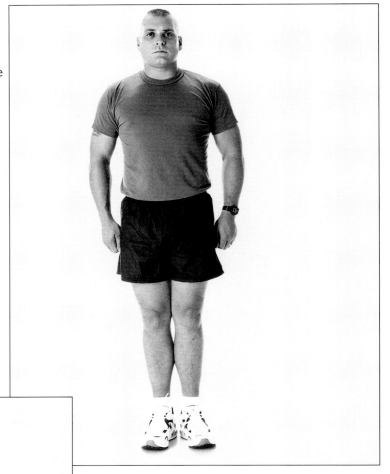

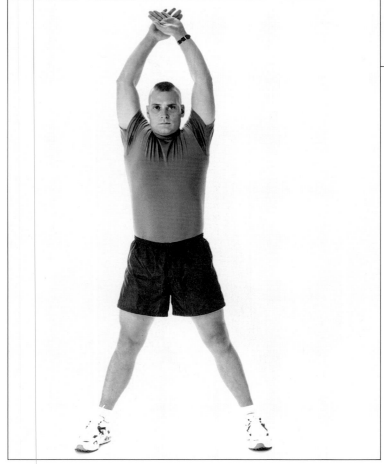

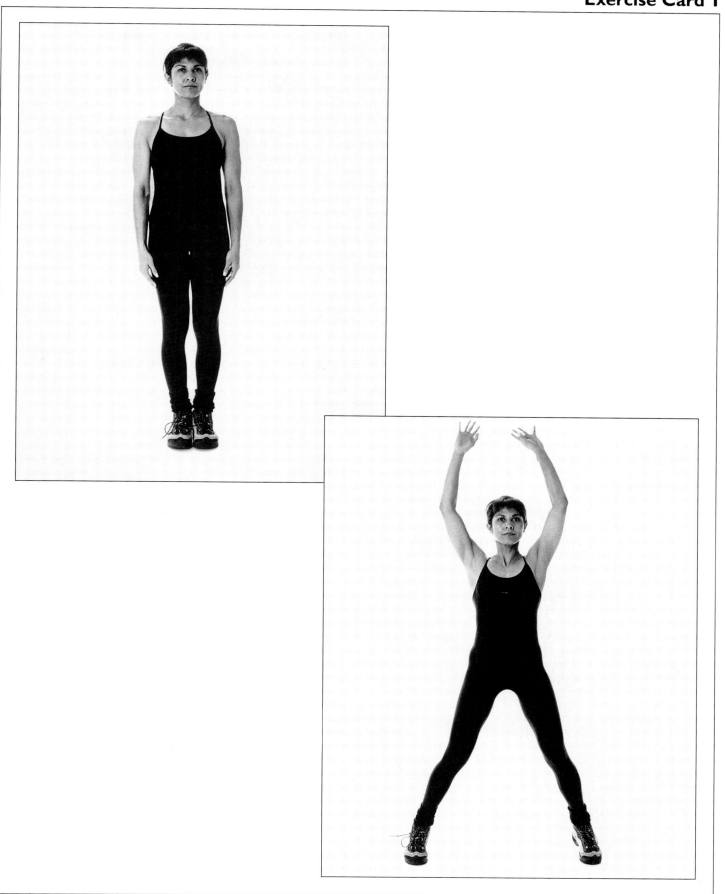

Exercise Card 2

Pushups
Crunches
Side leg raises
Diamond pushups
Elbow-to-knee crunches
Prone flutter kicks
Hip adduction
Lunges
Side straddle hops
Jack Webb

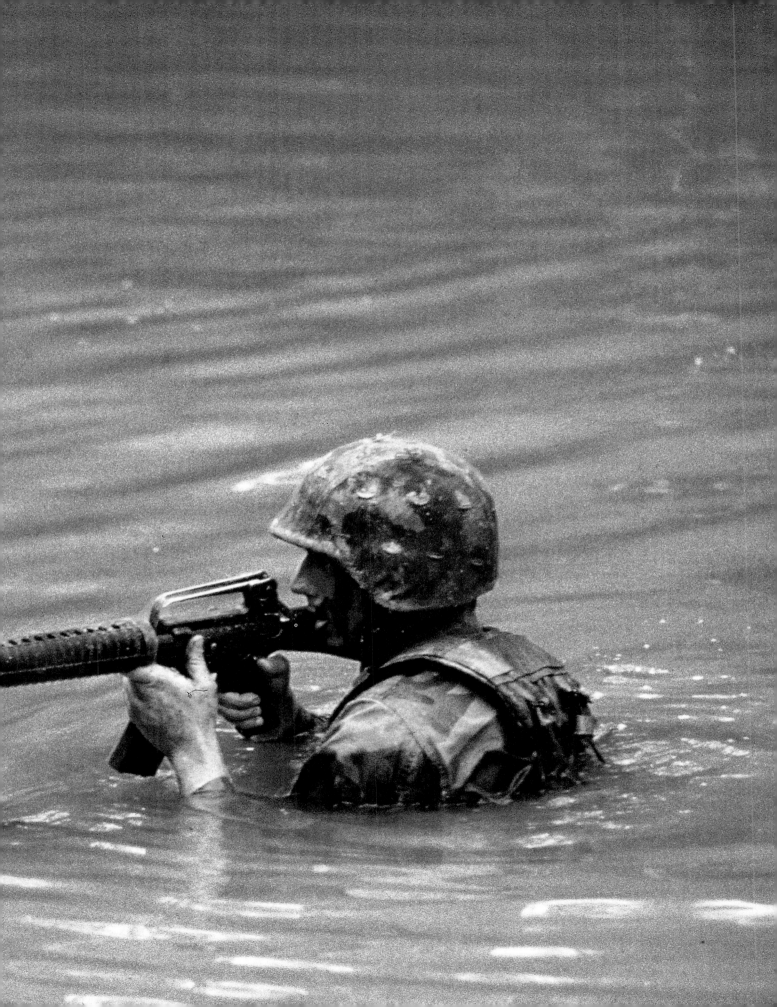

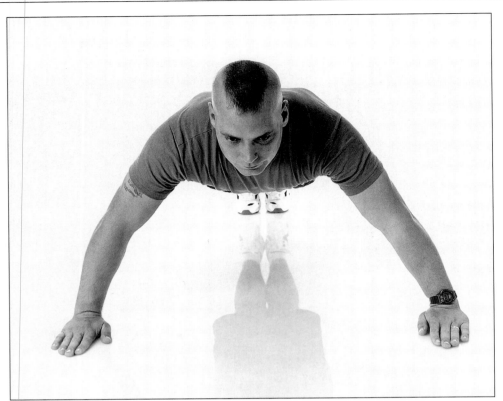

1. Pushups

Start with hands, shoulder width apart, and toes on the ground with elbows, back and knees straight.

On the first and third count, lower the chest to the deck, bending the elbows to at least 90 degrees.

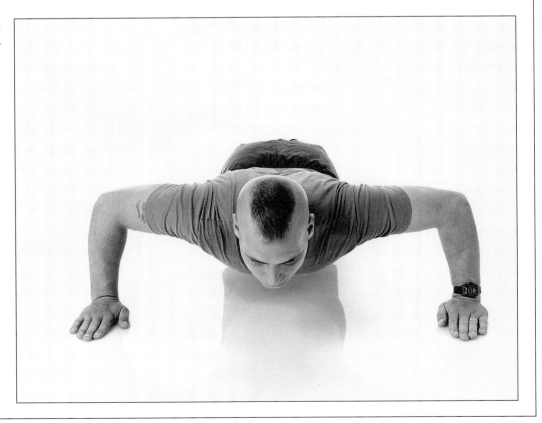

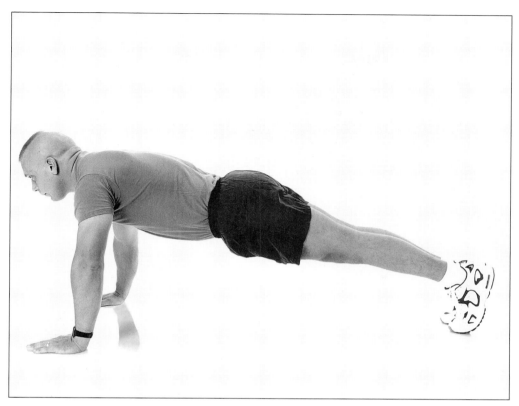

On the second and fourth count, extend the arms back to the starting position. This exercise primarily conditions the chest and anterior shoulder and, secondarily the triceps. Five to 10 repetitions.

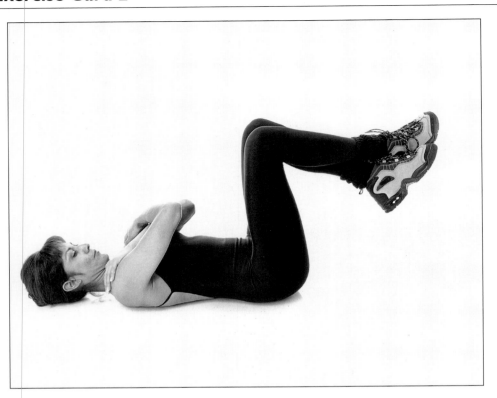

2. Crunches

Start on the back with hips bent to 90 degrees and knees bent, feet off the ground. Bend the elbows to 90 degrees and fold across the chest. On the first and third count, raise the upper torso off the deck, touching the thighs with the forearms. Make sure the chin remains on your chest. On the second and fourth count, return to the starting position. This should be one in a slow an controlled manner. This exercise conditions the abdominal muscles.
Five to 10 repetitions.

NOTE: When coming toward
the knees with the forearms,
it is not essential to make contact.
Come as close as you can.

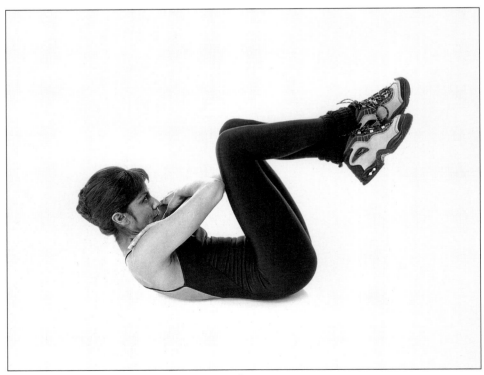

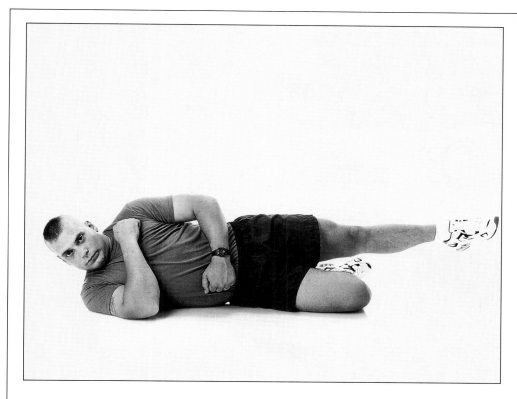

3. Side leg raises

Start on the right side with the right knee bent, the hip vertical, and the toes on the left foot pointing forward, *not to the sky*. On the first and third count, raise the left leg approximately 18 inches, leading with the heel. The toes will still point forward, *not to the sky*. On the second and fourth count, lower the right leg to the starting position. This exercise conditions the muscles on the side of the hip and thigh. Five to 10 repetitions.

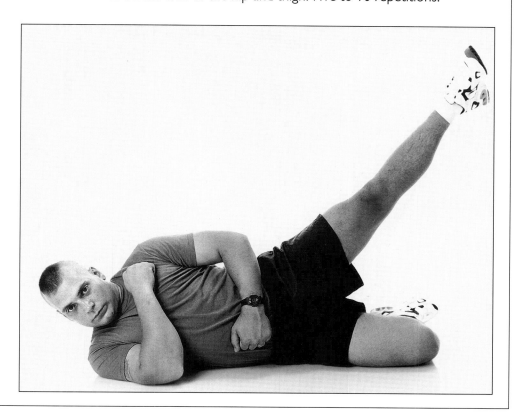

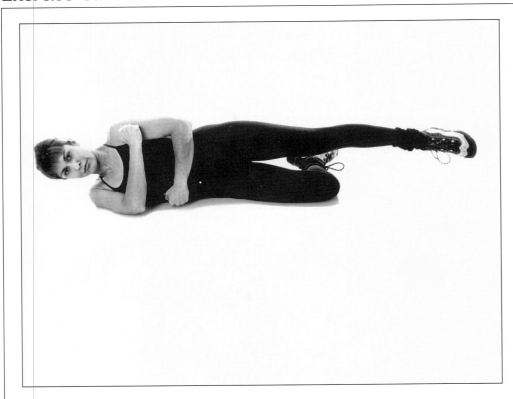

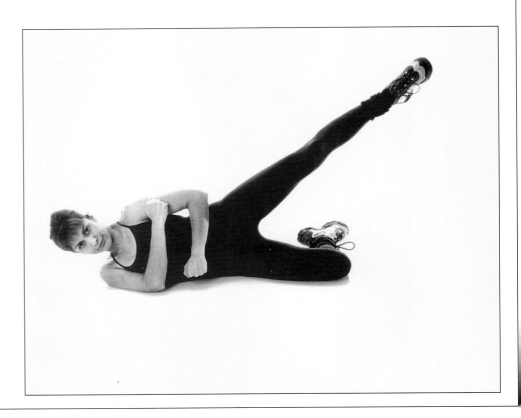

4. Diamond pushups

Assume a push-up position with the arms fully extended and the butt slightly raised. Form the fingers into a diamond shape by placing the forefinger and thumb of both hands together. On the count of one, lower the head as close as possible to the hands. Push back up until the arms are fully extended again in the starting position. Ten repetitions. This diamond pushup is a major triceps builder.

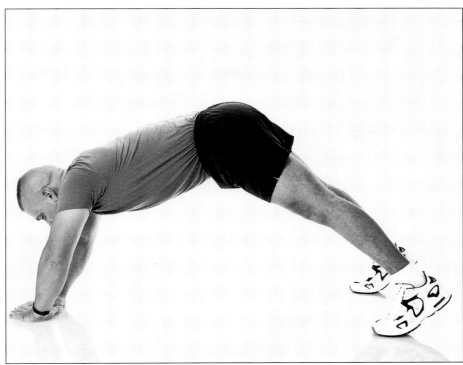

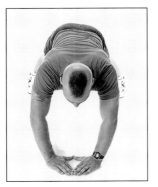

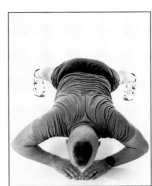

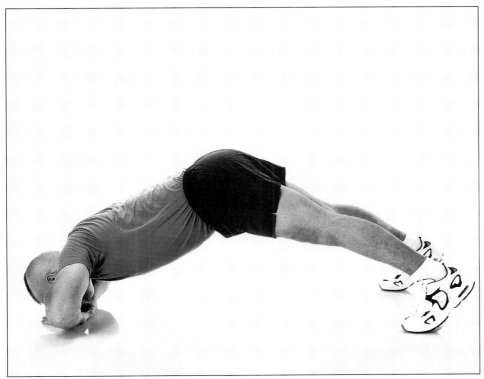

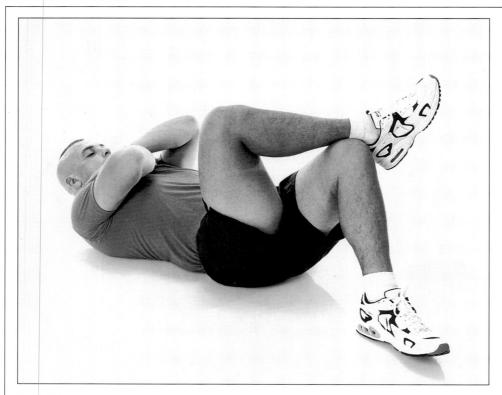

5. Elbow-to-knee crunches

Start with head and torso flat on the deck. The left foot is also flat on the deck and the right foot is crossed over the left knee. The arms are crossed on the chest. On the first and third count, raise the upper torso off the deck, rotating to the right, touching the left elbow to the right thigh. On the second and fourth count, return to the starting position. This should be done in a slow and controlled manner. Repeat to the other side. This exercise conditions the abdominal muscles with more emphasis on the obliques. Five to 10 repetitions.

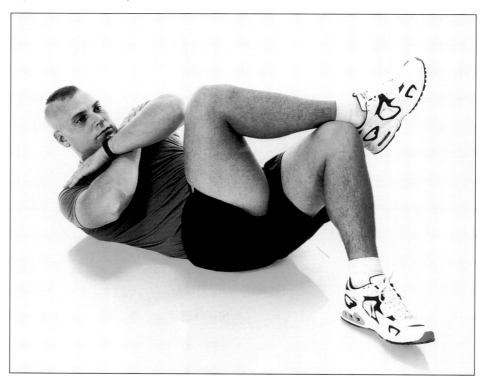

6. Prone flutter kicks

Start by lying on the stomach with hands extended, palms down, one palm over the other. On the first count, raise the left leg off the deck, keeping the right leg on the deck. On the second count, lower the left leg to the starting position. On the third count, raise the right leg off the deck keeping the left leg on the deck. On the fourth count, lower the right leg to the starting position. This exercise conditions the muscles that extend the hip and back. Five to 10 repetitions.

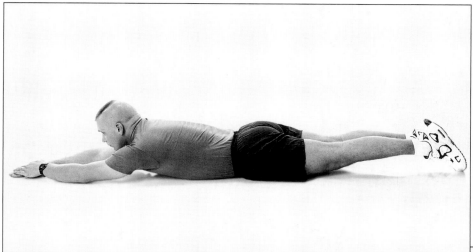

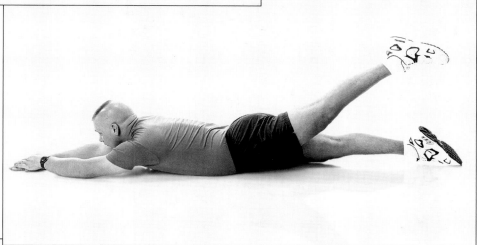

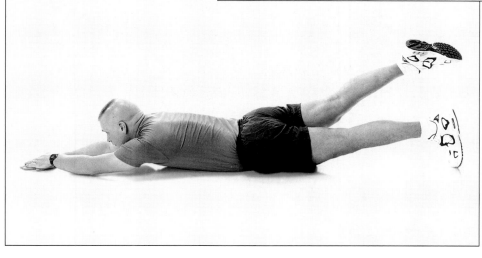

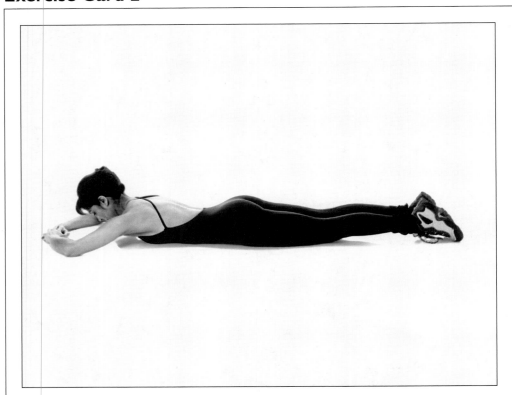

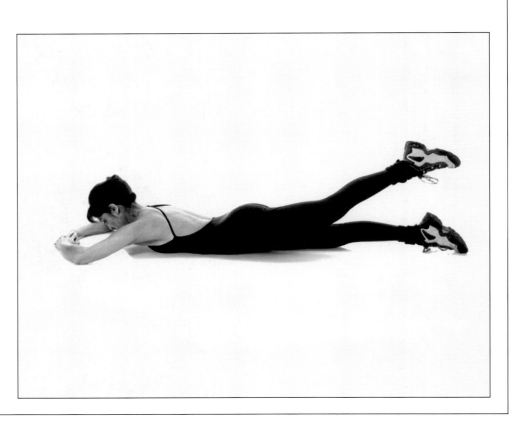

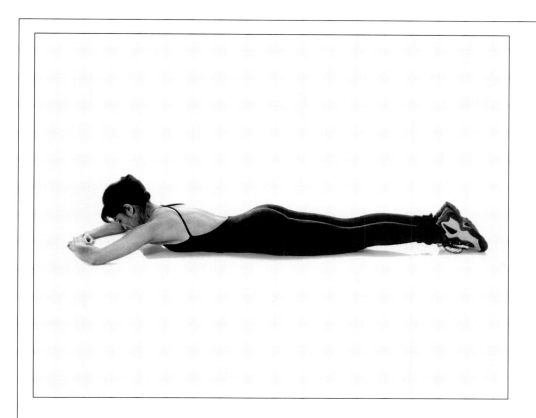

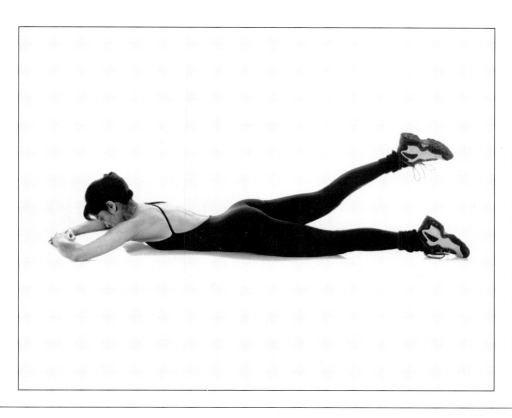

7. Hip adduction

Start on the right side with the left leg bent, setting the left foot in front of the right knee. On the first and third count, raise the straight right leg off the deck, squeezing the thighs together. On the second and fourth count, lower the right leg to the starting position. The right toes should be pointing straight forward, *not to the sky*. Repeat on the other side. This exercise conditions the muscles on the inner thigh. Five to 10 repetitions.

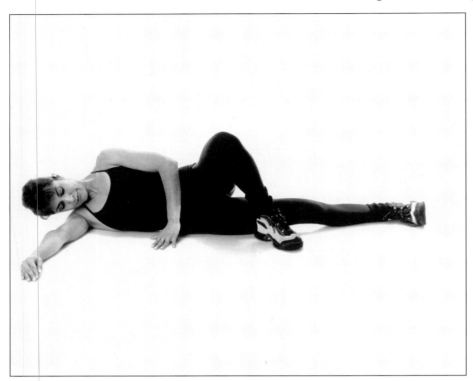

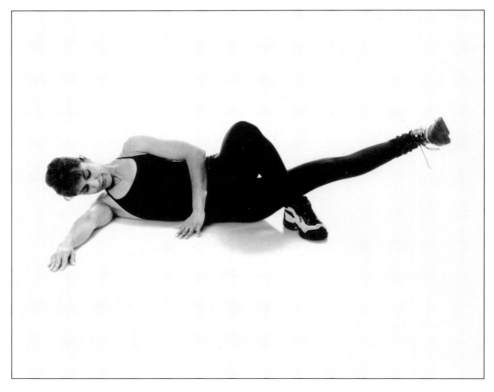

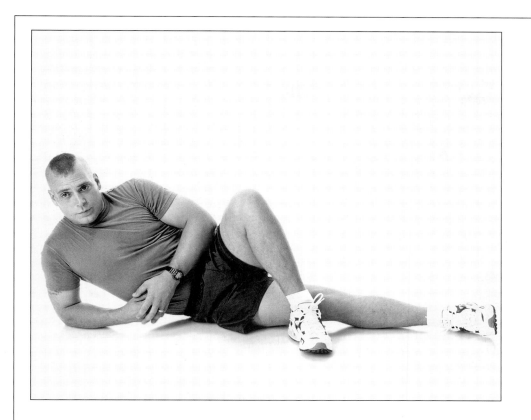

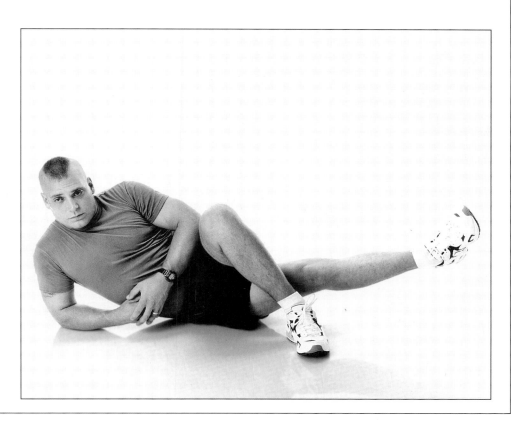

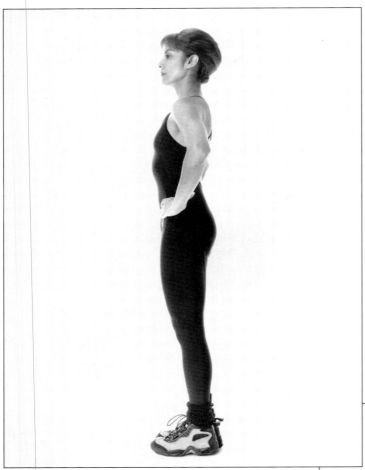

8. Lunges

Start standing with the feet shoulder-width apart and hands on the hips. On the first count, touch the right knee to the deck by stepping forward with the left foot and bending knees. On the second count, return to the starting position. On the third count, touch the left knee to the deck by stepping forward with the right foot and bending both knees. On the fourth count, return to the starting position. Do not bend the forward knee beyond the toes. Do in a controlled cadence. This exercise conditions the muscles that extend the hip and knee of the forward leg. Five to 10 repetitions.

NOTE: It is important to keep the back as straight as possible.

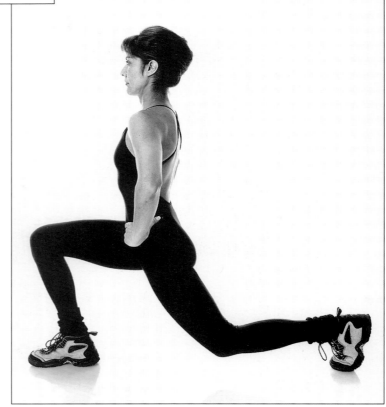

9. Side straddle hops

Stand erect with the feet together and arms at the sides. On the first and third count, jump and land with the feet just beyond shoulder width apart while bringing the hands together overhead. On the second and fourth count, jump back to the starting position. Five to 10 repetitions.

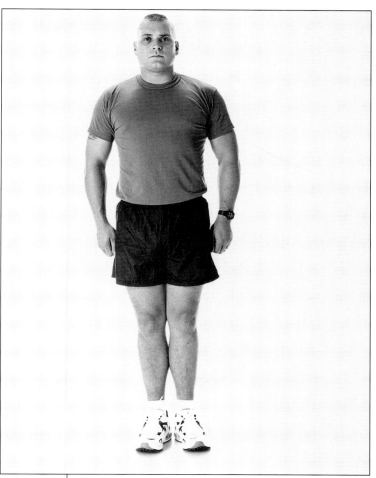

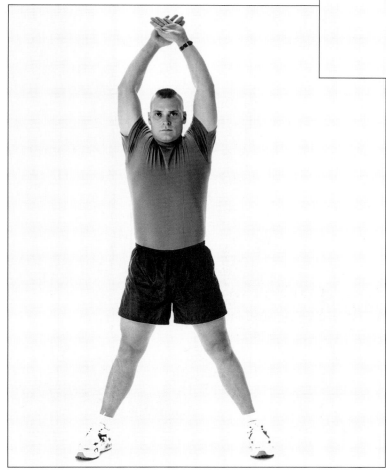

10. Jack Webb

This is a pyramid-style push up. Start in the prone push-up position and thrust the torso back, and bend the knees into the "prayer position" with the arms level to the shoulders. Then forcefully thrust both arms straight up. Then fall back down to the prone push-up position. Repeat until a set of five is completed. Once a set of five is completed, continue the repetitions while counting down from four to one.

NOTE: This is an advanced exercise and a good proof of upper body and triceps strength and endurance.

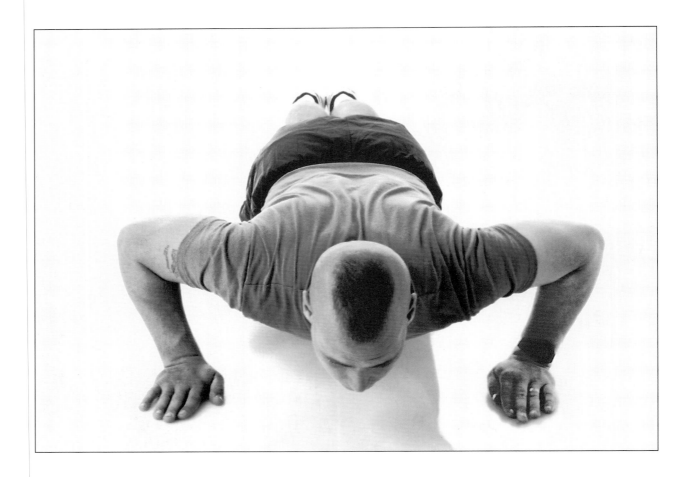

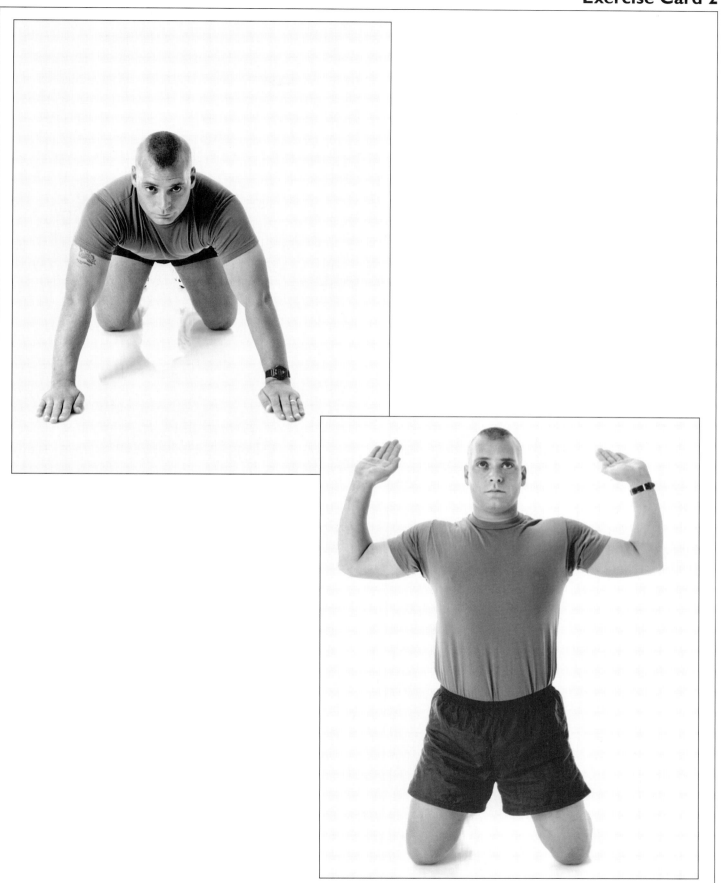

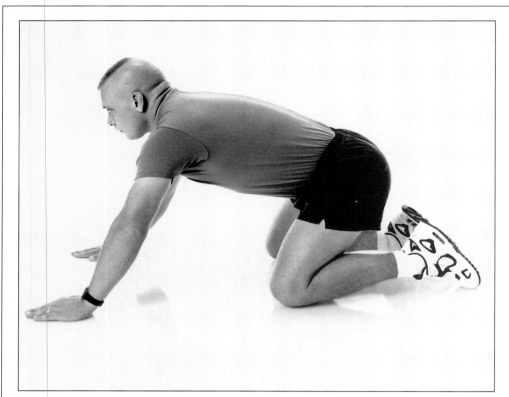

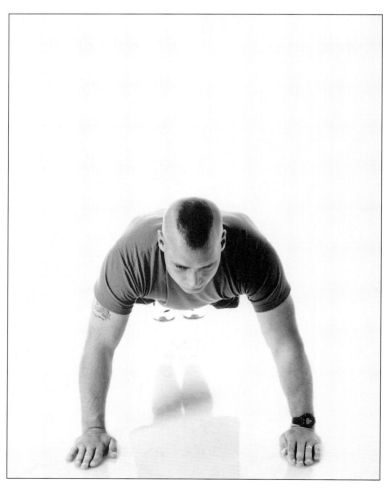

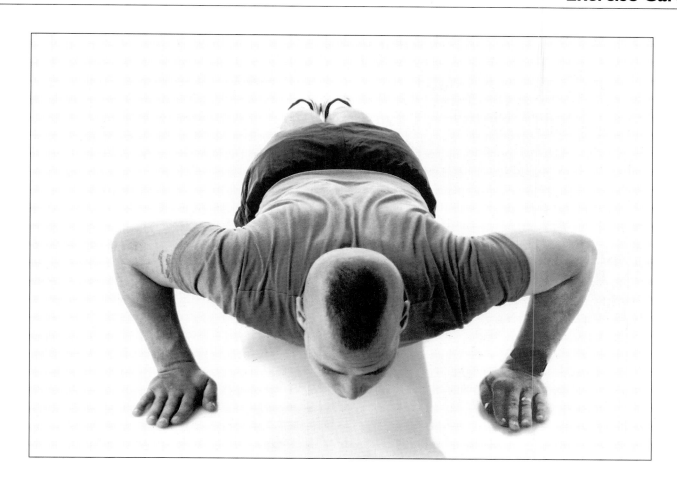

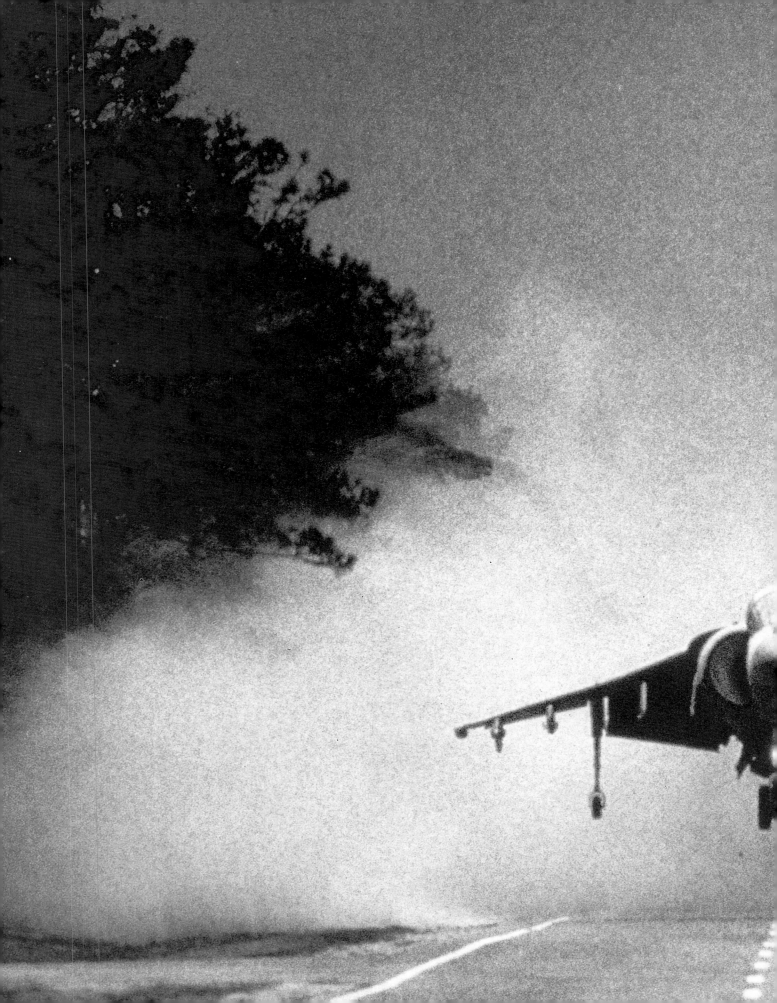

Marine Recruit Physical Training Test Requirements

MALE RECRUIT STANDARDS
3 mile run/28:00 min or less
pullups/8 or more
situps/50 or more

FEMALE RECRUIT STANDARDS
3 mile run/31:00 min or less
flex arm hang (FAH)/45 sec or more
situps/50 or more

Required minimal acceptable performance (male) for post-basic training semi-annual test

Age	Pullups	Situps	3-Mile Run
17-26	3	50	28:00 min.
27-39	3	45	29:00 min.
40-45	3	45	30:00 min.
46+	3	40	33:00 min.

Required minimal acceptable performance (female) for post-basic training semi-annual test

Age	FAH	Situps	3-Mile Run
17-26	15 sec.	50	31:00 min.
27-39	15 sec.	45	32:00 min.
40-45	15 sec.	45	33:00 min.
46+	15 sec.	40	36:00 min.

Bent knee situps

Time limit is two minutes for male and female Marines. In the correct starting position, participants are on their backs with their shoulder blades touching the deck, knees flexed, and both feet flat on the deck. The arms are folded across and remain against the chest or rib cage with no gap between the forearms and the chest or rib cage when raising the upper body. One repetition consists of raising the upper body from the starting position until the elbows or forearms touch the thighs and then returning the starting position with the shoulder blades touching the deck. No bouncing or arching of the lower back is authorized, and the buttocks will remain in constant contact with the deck throughout the exercise. An assistant may hold the feet or legs below the knees in whatever manner is most comfortable for the participants. Kneeling or sitting on the feet is permitted. Repeat as many times as possible during the time limit. Individuals may rest in either the up or down position.

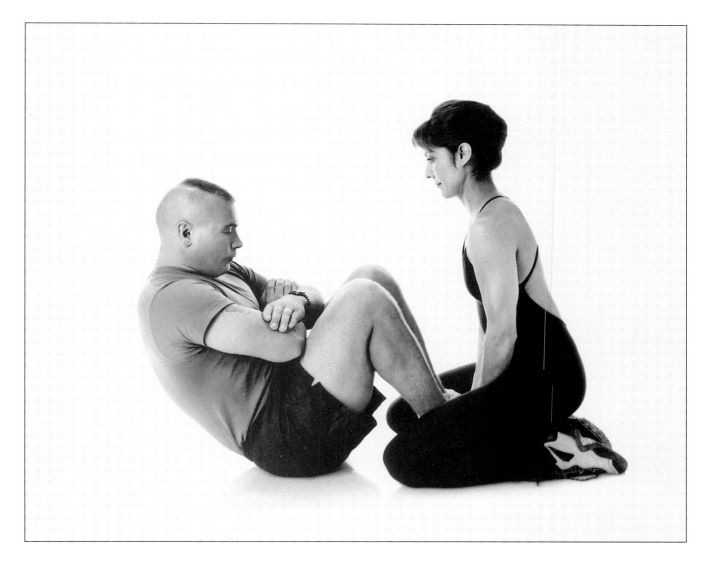

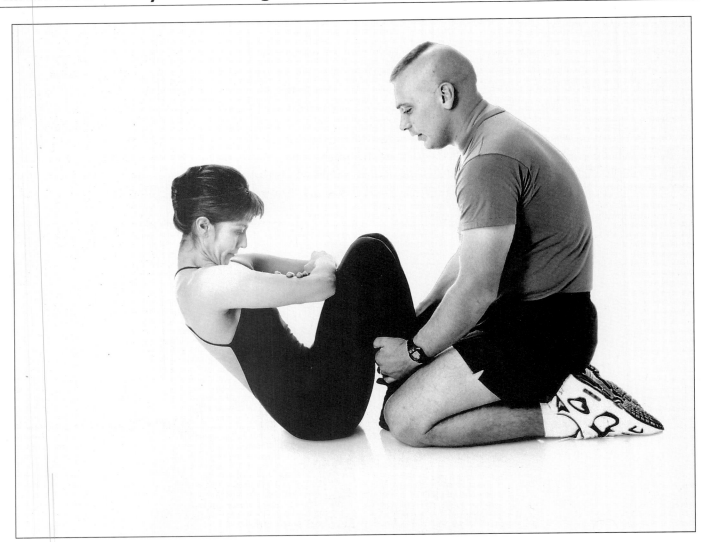

Pullups/Chinups (for males)

The participant may be assisted to the bar by a step up, by being lifted, or by jumping. The force of the jump will not be used to continue on into the first pullup/chinup. The bar is grasped with both palms facing either forward or to the rear; the arms are fully extended, and the feet are free of the ground. One repetition consists of raising the body with the arms until the chin is above the bar and lowering it until the arms are fully extended again. Repeat as many times as possible. Kicking motions such that the feet and/or knees do not raise above the waist level are permitted as long as the pullup remains a vertical movement. The body will be kept from swinging by an assistant holding an extended arm across the front of the knees of the Marine on the bar. Hand position may be changed during the exercise providing the individual does not dismount the bar or receive assistance from another party. Resting is permitted in the up or down position but resting with the chin supported by the bar is prohibited.

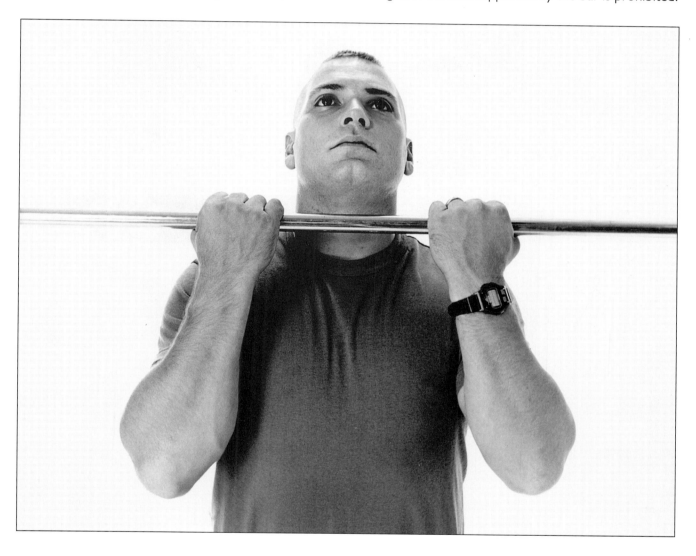

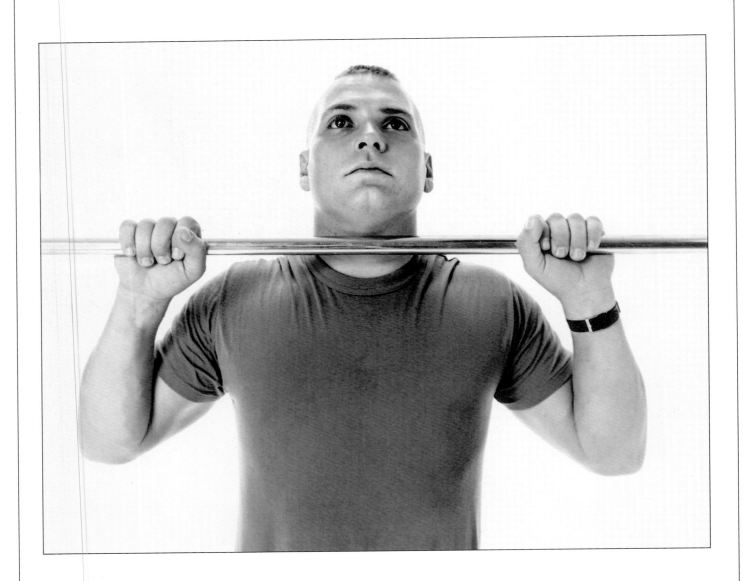

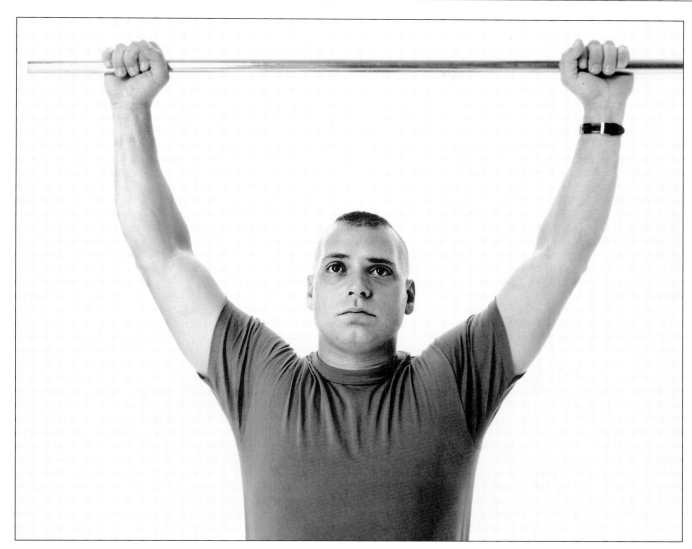

Pullups/Chinups (widespread position)

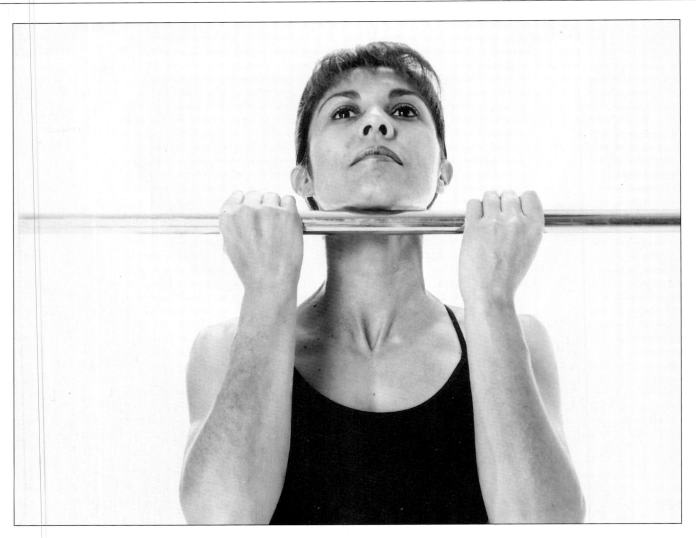

Flex arm hang (for females)

The individual jumps up or, if necessary, is assisted by others to reach the starting position. The bar may be grasped in any manner the individual desires, but both palms must face in the same direction. The elbows are flexed so that the chin is over or level with the bar. Once the individual is set in the starting position, the support or assistance is removed and she attempts to maintain elbow flexion for as long as possible. The score is the length in seconds that some degree of flexion at the elbow is maintained.